One Heart-Two Lives

Managing Your Rehabilitation Program WELL

Brent E. Zepke, Esq.

Brent E Zepke
3340 McCaw Avenue
Suite 207
Santa Barbara, CA. 93105
bezepke@gmail.com

ISBN: 0692462236
ISBN-13: 9780692462232

DEDICATION

To the powers that created this world and on January 10, 2007, gave me a second chance to continue to enjoy it,

To my wife, Carol Money Zepke, for making everyday a blessing,

To my children, Chad Eric, Hollie Anne and Grant Austin, for providing inspiration and incentive for my growth, and to their mother Anne Louise, for blessing me with her love and our children,

To my parents, June and George, for their sacrifices that I finally realized when I became a parent,

To the surgeons (Cisek, Westerman and West), cardiologist (Aragon), physicians (Ingersoll and the late Harry Flaster) nurses (Lynn Tabor and Jennifer Conger) and the other medical personnel of Sansum Clinic and Cottage Hospital, and the designers of all the machines, tests and medications that made my survival and rehabilitation possible,

To Mended Hearts, the cardiovascular peer-to-peer support network (mendedhearts.org), for helping me, and many others, progress through rehabilitation,

To Mike Kirsche for encouraging, editing and improving my manuscript as only a caring friend of over 60 years could, and

To Stan Eisele and my writing group for all their patience and assistance in shaping this book.

About the cover: It is the author and his wife walking past some feathered friends into the sunset on his "rehabilitation" beach.

Also by BRENT E. ZEPKE

Business Statistics

Products and the Consumer

Labor Law

Law for Non-Lawyers

Personnel Directors Legal Guide

Legal Guide to Human Resources

CONTENTS

CHAPTER 1. WEDNESDAY, JANUARY 10: THE END OF MY LIFE

On January 10, 2007, at 9:37 A.M. Pacific Time, my heart stopped. There were no pains in my chest, no dizziness, no blurred vision, no slurred speech, no pains in my jaw, no loss of hearing, no numbness of limbs, no gasping for breath, no bleeding, no strange tastes. At 9:36 A.M. I was sitting on the edge of a table with my legs swinging in front of me as I began a sentence with "I am headed to the YMCA for my daily workout of...." when my world disappeared. No flashes of light. No warning cries. No music. No heat. No cold. No smells. No tastes. No feelings. No comfort. No discomfort. No thoughts. No dreams. No fears. No joys. No regrets. No anticipations. No white lights. No "why me?" or "why now?" No flashing of people from my past. No happiness. No sadness. No pulse. No vital functions. No anything. No life.

Time was the enemy of any hope of my defying the odds that for 97 of every 100 people whose heart stops, these would be the last words ever passing through my now limp lips. Even before the head of my now limp body hit the cinderblock wall, time had started running against it. At 9:37 A.M., everything about time changed. Time, which for over sixty three years had been celebrated by the number of years lived, was put on super fast forward. Time was no longer counted in years, months, weeks, days, not even in hours, but minutes and every one of the sixty seconds in each one. Each tick of the second hand of the clock on the wall reduced my chances of joining the other 2 in 100 who would be recalled to life. For the chosen few who would return, time was even shorter for preventing brain damage: after 3-5 minutes with no oxygen the risks became extremely high. Each tick-tock raised the chances of brain damage. After five minutes, there would be a greater risk of not being recalled to life. In 7 minutes it was almost a certainty that no one, including me, would be recalled to life.

The "me" was a six foot, 205 pound, 63 plus year old male who had every reason to think he was in good health. Three hours and thirty-seven minutes earlier on this 10th day of January, I was awakened by the alarm signaling it was time for me to begin what I thought was a normal day. I made breakfast for my wife Carol before she went to work. I had become the designated breakfast maker after my retirement from practicing law. Notice I said "breakfast maker" because my preparing coffee and oatmeal would not qualify me as a chef. After breakfast, my typical day was studying the stock market, cleaning the kitchen and writing something for my writing class; all while thinking of my children. Our living in Santa Barbara, California, had many advantages and one major disadvantage: it was too expensive for my children. My son Chad lived in Delaware, my daughter Hollie, in Seattle, and my other son, Grant, in North Carolina.

On this January 10th, I woke up feeling the same as I did pretty much every morning: no aches, no pains. Carol headed for the shower while in my semi-daze I started the coffee and heated the water for the oatmeal we ate almost every morning, as part of our efforts to live a long, healthy life. Our breakfast was not the type featured in so many movies of sitting by a pool while a server presented a spectacular breakfast. In our case, after I served breakfast we sat in bed balancing the bowls in our laps with Investors' Business Daily and the Wall Street Journal, half listening to the talking heads on CNBC. Such is the breakfast of an investor: efficient, yes; relaxing, no. This has been our routine for over five years. An unexpected consequence of being in Santa Barbara, California, was that the New York Stock Exchange, which opens at 9:30 Eastern Time, opens at 6:30 A.M. Pacific Time, forcing an early start, and closed at 1 P.M., freeing up the entire afternoon.

This morning, as I cleaned the kitchen, I thought of how strange it still seemed that, after 30 years of practicing law, I no longer entered my closet every week day morning to select the tie that would best go with my dark suit of the day. I was as much a perfectionist in my appearance as I was in the rest of my life: the color of the design in my tie had to match my shirt; my cuff links had to be carefully aligned and my belt must match my shoes, which were always brightly polished ever since I had read that polished shoes defined a well dressed man. However, on this day, as with all the other mornings since my job had been eliminated as a result of the attack on the twin towers on 9/11, my suit was replaced by exercise shorts and a sweat shirt and my highly polished shoes by sneakers; I was headed for the YMCA after I completed my routine stress echo test. I say "routine" because for years during my annual physical it was recommended that I get a follow up stress echo test, which I always passed. My recent one, a year ago to the day, had ended with the cardiologist saying "Have a good life." During the early summer, my annual physical had shown no reason to doubt I was in good health. In anticipation of starting a diet, the ever cautious me had seen my physician for blood work. On my next visit, my physician had entered the examination room smiling and shook my hand saying, "Congratulations, your blood work is great."

The only unusual aspect of this January 10th, which at the time I didn't give much thought, was when Carol asked, "Would you like me to go with you for your test?" I confess to being a little surprised since we never accompany each other unless one of us thinks it may be serious. Without giving much thought as to whether this was a premonition, I resorted to my east coast humor and said, "No but you might consider taking out life insurance for me for at least this morning." You can bet this was the last time I will ever say that!

On many mornings at 7:45 AM., both Carol and I would drive our cars one block to the corner where our street, McCaw Avenue, dead ends into Las Positas Avenue. Carol would turn left towards her downtown office and I would turn right towards what I euphemistically refer to my western office; which actually was a chair on the beach at the Pacific Ocean, where I would study Investor's Business Daily. Many times on these days I would think of the story Al McGuire would tell about his days as the basketball coach of Marquette University in Milwaukee. He would say, "Each day the decision at my corner gets tougher: should I turn left to downtown and work, or right to the mountains and play."

On this January 10th, I was leaving a little later as my test was scheduled for 9 A.M. During the past year, I had followed the rules by getting clearance from my doctors before increasing my exercise program to reduce the tiredness that I attributed to either being somewhat out-of-shape or having never been this age before, or both. During my three trips a week to the YMCA I had gradually increased my time on the cardio machines. I particularly liked the elliptical machine with the handles where I could monitor my heart rate. I did have some confusion as to the maximum rate applicable to me. For my age, the charts listed it as both 140 beats per minute and a target rate of 85% above my resting heart rate; which at 64 beats per minute meant a target of 118. Should I use 140 or 118? I decided to compromise and use 130 because I sometimes experienced tightness in my chest around that number. It was not a pain. I was not certain what it was but I relied on medical reports that indicated no heart problems. But out of caution, if it persisted after I slowed down, I would get off the machine and call it a day. I did have some moments when I questioned whether my shortness of breath was only because of my age and weight, like the time I had to stop and catch my breath while walking up a hill at Yosemite Park. When Carol saw this she urged me to visit Urgent Care, where the physician did not detect any problems, but recommended that I move up my scheduled January appointment for a stress test. I agreed but on the scheduled date, December 6, 2006, my 12-year old Jaguar refused to start, so my test was rescheduled for January 10, 2007; a year to the day since my previous stress tests.

On this day, my Jaguar started and I turned left at the corner for my two mile ride to the clinic for my routine stress test. "Routine" because this has been an annual event for the ten years since my electrocardiogram (EKG) tests, a part of my annual physical, began showing an abnormality. The EKG is an inexpensive, non-intrusive (meaning it does not involve a penetration of the skin) test to identify abnormalities in the electrical activity of the heart. The EKG has a relatively high rate of false positives; i.e., indicating a problem where there is not one. At my former employer, so many people flunked the EKG that we thought the nurse was not administering the test properly. Subsequently, physicians have told me I have a harmless thickness in my

4

heart wall.

When I would flunk an EKG, or more scientifically stated "an abnormality was identified," I was referred to a cardiologist for a more expensive, precise test. Sometimes the referral was for an angiogram, which is an intrusive test where a tube is inserted in a patient's vein and threaded to the heart, where a tiny camera permits the physician to view the heart. A less intrusive test, the one I am scheduled for today, is a stress echo test. A "stress echo test" is the abbreviation for a "stress electrocardiogram" (ECG). The procedure is to attach electrodes to the patient to measure the blood flow through their heart at rest, then at stress and then the time it takes to come to rest again. "Stressed" is a polite term for forcing the heart to beat faster through the use of a treadmill. The entire process is recorded and displayed on a screen as it occurs.

On this January 10th, I took the slow elevator to the third floor of the clinic. As I entered the waiting room, I was tracked by many pairs of eyes peeking over the top of their magazines. Answering the questions about my medical history was always easy: a straight set of "no's" as my last surgery had been as a boy when I had my tonsils removed. Attached was a consent form. My legal training had taught me that these forms were used as a legal defense if a problem arose, by showing that the patient had "voluntarily assumed the risks;" a phrase that indicates a defense if it can be proved. One time, I inadvertently tested the importance of signing this form. It occurred when they were preparing my infant son Chad for surgery. I agreed to sign the form only after crossing out that we had been advised of the risks since we had not. An emotional scene escalated when a nurse threatened to cancel the surgery. The nurse stormed but returned with the surgeon, who explained the risks. I signed and the surgery was a success.

On this January 10th, I signed the form for the stress test without being advised of the risks. A woman in a light green gown led me down a hall, through a right turn and down the short light green hallway to the last examination room on the left. This room, like all the others, was a square approximately 12 feet by 12 feet. The sun was peaking in through the closed blinds of the only window. On my immediate right was a treadmill against the wall. Straight ahead was an examination table. There was a computer sitting on a table with wires connected to electrodes.

As I was being prepared, it became obvious that today my test was going to be conducted by a trainee who would take directions from the lead technician standing behind her. My cardiologist said "hello," before leaving and not returning during the test; perhaps because of the statistic that, in medical terms, only one stress test taker in every 100,000 has a seriously "negative" outcome from the test. The technician attached electrodes in multiple places on my chest, stomach and arms, while telling me to relax. I wondered how many people were able to really relax with electrodes from a computer attached by wires to their bodies.

I stood with the wires hanging off me while the technicians established a base line. Most peoples' normal resting heart rate is between 60 and 90 beats per minute. The technician said "Your heart rate of 60 beats per minute is typical of athletes," which helped my confidence.

I stepped on the treadmill and the speed and elevation were gradually increased to "stress" my heart rate, under medically controlled conditions, to a prescribed multiple of my resting rate. As my walking became more difficult, I worried about the same slight, strange feeling in the left side of my chest that I have had at the YMCA. But I thought it must be alright as they were monitoring me on the computer through the electrodes connected to my chest. My sweating increased, but I was not overly concerned because I always sweat when exercising. I asked myself, "had it gotten warmer in here?" I thought that it must be nerves. I pushed on; determined not to repeat the test of several years ago that was stopped prematurely based on my casual question of "how am I doing?" My cardiologists subsequently told me stopping the test ruined its validity.

The treadmill stopped and I was rushed to the examination table so they could continue the measurements while my heart started to slow down or, in medical terms "recovered." I have previously been told my recovery times are very quick. As instructed, I laid on my left side with my legs drawn up while gasping for air. But the test was designed to force gasping. When I took in a breath, the trainee said, "Hold it in." Not taking a breath while gasping for air was difficult. But it was nowhere near as difficult as her next direction of "don't take a breath" after I had left the last one out. After what seemed like an eternity, she repeated "don't take a breath" while asking the lead technician "which switch do I turn?" I started to lose consciousness, and involuntarily gasped for air.

At the five minute mark for the scheduled six minute rest period, I was permitted to sit up on the edge of the table. I was relieved the test was over. My heavy breathing was quickly subsiding. I was fully confident that I had passed since the computer's showing any problems would have stopped the test. My cardiologist entered the room and, while standing so close our knees almost touched, said to the technician "You can start taking the electrodes off" (*). I started telling the cardiologist about my exercise program until, mid-sentence, I stopped talking. The cardiologist said nothing. The technician said, "Are you all right?"

No words came from my mouth. The technician asked again. I did not respond. When the technician leaned back to look at my face, he saw the pupils of my eyes "roll up and disappear." My limp body collapsed backwards in a free fall. He grabbed for me but my now limp body twisted and my forehead hit the wall hard. I never felt it. My heart had stopped beating. I had defied the odds: I had become the one in 100,000 suffering a major "negative" event during this test. The odds now were 97 to 3 against my returning to life. Using the medical term of "flat lining," of every 100 flat liners, 3 return. For the other 97 this is their demise, expiration, end, exit, passage, passing, quietus from life. Their vital functions stop forever. Their time on earth is over. When my heart, after beating for sixty three years, two hundred eighty eight days and ten minutes, stopped: I had become a flat liner!

(*) All conversations in this book represent my best recollections.

CHAPTER 2. THE BEGINNING OF MY LIFE

I was a middle child born into a world of stress: wars and depressions can have that effect on families. On the very Sunday of my birth in 1943, during World War II, while my German descent father was helping his British descent wife, my mother, through labor; a thousand miles away the German commander of the submarine U-159 was sinking the British ship Silverfish. Much as the sailors of the Silverfish were being sunk by the war, so were the plans of my parents. On the very next day as my parents were marveling at my full head of brown hair, the war was creeping further into their room at West Jersey Hospital. They quickly learned that their plans for bringing me home by stretching the war time ration of four gallons of gasoline a week was only the beginning of the stretching necessary for families as that very day the rationing was being extended by the addition of meat, butter and bread, to the existing rations list of shoes, sugar, tires, silk, nylons and, of course, gasoline. Sixty years later tears ran out of the corners of my mother's eyes when she said, "I remember standing in line with my coupon book hoping there would be some meat left."

For centuries wars have added stress to families, and mine was no exception. At the age of five my paternal grandfather's family brought their son, John Zepke, from Germany to Oaklyn, New Jersey, where he would marry an Irish lady, Elizabeth Brady. They were so proud of their country that they named their first, and only, son "George Washington" Zepke. While my father was starting school, John worked making ships to fight the country of his birth, Germany, in World War I. When my father was nine, the death of his mother caused him to take responsibility for helping to raise his three-year old sister Jean. They remained close in feelings and geography for their entire lives.

My maternal grandfather, of British descent, had been named "Grover Cleveland" Stackhouse after the American President who had the unusual distinction of serving both as the 22nd and 24th president. Grover married Ellen MacDonald, of Scottish descent, and in 1918, on the eve of the Battle of Amiens in World War I, gave birth to my mother, June Stackhouse, and two years later her only sibling, her sister Eleanor. My mother would reminisce about hearing the sounds of the bells on horses pulling wagon with the driver yelling "ice for sale" as there were no refrigerators, or her mother saying "girls it is time for your bath," as she poured pots of water, heated on the stove, into a tub in the kitchen for her sister and her, then her mother and finally her father.

Both my parents were proud of being the first in their families to graduate from an American high school. My father in 1929, at the start of the Great Depression, and my mother, in 1933, right into the Depression that lasted until the start of World War II in 1941. Their aspirations to go to college and become an engineer (father) and teacher, derailed by their needing to immediately help support their families, were transferred to their children. Like wars, depressions can be tough and this one was so tough it was labeled the "Great Depression." Unemployment rose to 24% in 1932, and averaged 19.5% until the U.S. entered World War II in 1941. My mother remembers a foreman standing on a loading dock of the Campbell's Soup Company and telling the crowd of job seekers, "Anyone not willing to work for a dollar an hour can leave," followed by, "Anyone who will not work for seventy five cents an hour can leave." At whatever the rate was when the crowd dwindled down to the number of workers needed, became the starting rate."

Anyone fortunate enough, like my father, to obtain employment tried to do things "perfectly" in order to keep it. This standard had a special meaning for my father as he began his 42 year career at DuPont in a laboratory where he had to decide whether to accept, or reject, tanks filled with hundreds of gallons of paint. To ensure consistency he learned to be very precise in his actions and unwavering in his conclusions; both of which qualities he also applied to his family. Tears formed in my usually non-emotional mother's eyes when, at 93, she said "If you have ever lived through depression, you will never forget it."

A few years before my birth my parents finally felt secure enough to give birth to my brother Barry. Just a few months later, on December 7, 1941, the Japanese bombing Pearl Harbor blew my parents' security apart. As the U.S. entered World War II, my father's expertise in making finishes for military vehicles prevented his enlisting in the military but not from DuPont's freezing his wages and, ultimately, his career. After the war ended, as the U.S. rebuilt the countries that had caused the war---Japan and Germany---and the returning veterans entered college on the G.I Bill, wages at DuPont remained so low that thirty years later my father's voice broke when he told me about the man next to him who, when told his long promised raise was a penny an hour, said "You can take this job and shove it."

My father's need to continue to support his family kept him from doing the same. The steady employment was good and bad: good because he could support his family, and bad because later they put him on rotating shifts that destroyed his hopes of night school, his beloved bowling leagues, and, eventually, his marriage.

My father was stern, often very stern, but not a bad man. He was well intended but wars and depressions had created a life time of quiet, and sometimes not so quiet, desperation. He always felt that in order to support his family his every action had to be "perfect." At work this produced sufficient results to propel him through to retirement, but at home it led to his judging our activities as always being able to have "done it better" without any suggestions of "how." I never remember receiving even a "well done" from him.

My brother Barry and I entered school just before the Korean War and during this war the birth of my sister Jill completed our family. After a childhood full of dinners listening to my father's frustrations at being frozen in place while non-performing college educated engineers were promoted, we three planned on attending college. At the end of my sophomore year in high school my brother's accident in the family car exposed a sad fact. All the years of my parents' assuring him, and me, that they were saving for our college that night proved it was not true. At sixteen I learned my parents had been telling us untruths!

This revelation was life changing. If I could not rely on the words of my parents, then whose words or promises could I rely on? I still remember sitting night after night at the desk by the front window in the bedroom in Haddonfield, New Jersey, I shared with my brother as my feelings slowly transitioned through hopelessness to determination. Even over fifty years later I vividly remember watching the salesman next door drive off to Virginia, the attorney with the homburg hat and news paper tucked under his arm walk to the bus stop for daytime jobs. I came to see that in the world outside my window there were people of my parents' generation who had overcome the same wars and depressions that had limited my parents. How that transition in my attitude occurred remains a mystery to me, since we did not take a newspaper, never watched the news on television, the creators of the Internet would not be born for another thirty years and my friends and neighbors were no different. But somehow I decided that our governing documents meant that there were opportunities "out there" to create the life style I sought. I just had to obtain the education necessary to earn it.

I greatly respected my parents, whose values had been formed during times of horse drawn ice wagons and bath water heated on wood burning stoves, for sacrificing their hopes and dreams in order to raise a family through wars and a depression. I knew they could not financially help me, not because of a lack of desire but because of a lack of resources. I was bothered by their misleading me on their ability to financially help me, but my thoughts slowly shifted being wishing they had been able to offer more emotional support to me and to have had more pleasures in their lives. I related to my father when the father of a friend, a navy captain, said "The hardest thing you will ever do is go to work every day."

At sixteen, in many ways I became a man. A man full of the enthusiasm of youth and the ambitions of a dreamer who had no idea how to proceed except through the classroom. Not being able to rely on the words of my parents stimulated many of my core values, such as taking responsibility for myself and my actions, my word being my bond and the words of others were just empty words without consistent actions. The view through my window showed me that some other people had created a better life style. I developed a saying I still use for inspiration: no one was born knowing their professions, so each skill is a learned one, and if someone else could learn it, then so can I."

Years later my friend, the singer Jim Morris, and I created the appropriate phrase of "Creativity is directly related to desperation." And desperate I was: so I got busy. I decided that the ages from 18-25 would determine the quality of the rest of my life so I decided to skip any of the "distractions" that others my age were enjoying, such as new cars and fun filled evenings. I also got lucky: I fell in love in high school with a classmate Anne Whitaker, who would emotionally support me for 25 years while all others, including hers and my parents, did not.

By a combination of scholarships and working any job I could find, like night work in a paint factory, a cashier in a food store, a file clerk, a clothing salesman at Sears, a customer engineer at IBM, a truck loader at UPS, and teaching shop math and then industrial engineering, I was able to finance, and earn, a bachelor's degree in mathematics from the University of North Carolina and a masters degree in Industrial Management from Clemson University. When the University of Tennessee hired me to teach statistics, I used the opportunity to have both a full time teaching load and be a full time law student. Once my then wife Anne carried me through some of the inevitable dark days accompanying being both a full time faculty member and law student. In my third year of law school as we were blessed with the birth of my son Chad, my teaching shifted to production management, organizational management, business policy and while studying for the bar exam business law. After graduating, as I started a position in the law department of Gulf Oil Corporation, we were blessed with a daughter, Hollie, and son, Grant. Life was good.

When I was in my thirties, a conversation occurred that summarized my childhood relationship with my father. When he followed his practice of ignoring my opinion, something in me snapped and I said, "You really are stubborn."

He responded, "I am not stubborn, I am determined."

I was surprised that he obviously had thought this through and prepared his answer, so I said, 'What's the difference?"

With a smile he said, "A stubborn person takes a position and never changes because he took it. A determined person takes a position and never changes because he is right."

In the summer of 1981, my life had settled in to what I thought of as "normal."

CHAPTER 3. RECALLED TO LIFE

On January 10, 2007, my heart stopping instantly eliminated all indications of life. Even the cardiologist standing two feet away never had any doubts: life had left what used to be my body. Breathing, thinking, moving, talking, listening, and every other function associated with being alive disappeared. The body that I had occupied for over sixty three years had become a "dead weight," not lying as a living being but laying in a crumpled mass, as an inanimate object, on a table in a small room on the third floor of a clinic in California.

"Sudden cardiac arrests" can have that effect. Scientists will say that my brain was the first part of my body to suffer. It does not store any blood, so any interruption of the blood flow immediately stops it from functioning. My brain stopping shut down any ability to process input from my eyes, ears, nose, and hands or from any other parts of my nervous system. To the untrained eye, the symptoms could indicate unconsciousness. Unconsciousness means "lacking awareness and the capacity for sensory perception" (the free dictionary), including not responding to loud sounds or shaking (Health Line). To the untrained eye the initial symptoms of unconsciousness and flat lining (to register on an electronic monitor as having no brain waves or heart beat) may appear to be the same, but not to the medical community. These folks know that in unconsciousness the body continues to function; in flat lining it does not. Combating unconsciousness occurs almost all the time: combating flat lining almost never occurs. The question was not whether life had left that body: it had. The question was whether it could, or would, return.

Where was my spirit? I was not aware of being on the table or in the room or in the clinic but I was also not aware of being anywhere else. I was just not aware; not of any place, person or thing. I was not aware of my head hitting the wall or of any pain. It was not like an out-of-body experience where you see your body from outside it. I didn't see it or anything else. I was not aware that my eyes, ears, nose and every other part of my body no longer worked. I was not aware of leaving this world, or of staying in it. All thoughts of today, tomorrows or yesterdays stopped. The body that I had occupied just laid on the table. When my brain stopped, did I stay in the body or go somewhere? Who or what was I? Was there even a me?

I had no flashbacks, no streaming videos of my past, present or future; no sense of movement up or down; no anything. Where was I? Were these things occurring but I was just unaware of them? Time ceased to matter to me, but it became the enemy to any hopes of survival. Did some force greater than me decide that I could defy the 97 to 3 odds against being recalled to life? If the decision took five minutes or longer, I most likely would have brain damage. If the decision took at least seven minutes, the odds were almost 100% of my joining the 97 of every 100 who do not survive sudden cardiac arrest. After ten minutes, it was a certainty. The odds were stacked against me!

I only had two things in my favor. One was the location I was in was practically the only location where I could survive: a cardiology department. The other reason was that my otherwise good health gave me the power to be able to respond to the help from a force greater than me that had decided that it was not my time. Why? Did that force have something in mind for me? Was part of the reason I was here still undone? I can't answer any of these but I can say that I won the greatest lottery imaginable: I won life! I was recalled to life. I was given a second chance at life. My time between lives was short enough that there was no brain damage, but I have been too superstitious to ask the exact time.

I was oblivious to all these thoughts as I began my second life on the tenth day of January, 2007. My first indication that my second life had begun was the sound of a voice. Hearing was only possible after blood had again started being pumped to my brain, which meant my heart was working again. But at that time all I knew was a gradual awareness of a voice. It was vague, more like a hum without words. But I was aware. I was alive. I would love to say that when I became aware I was able to identify where I had been; but I cannot. It was, and is, a blank. I would love to say that on my return I could feel my heart beat, or my blood rush through my carotid arteries to restart my brain; but I cannot. I would like to say I immediately asked what happened; but I did not. I would like to say that I got up and walked out of the clinic; but I did not. I can say I became aware of something moist being pressed against my forehead. I can say I was able to open my eyes and see a relative clear image of a blond lady leaning over me and pressing a moist cloth on my forehead with her right hand. I had no thoughts of who she was, or why she was leaning over me, but I knew it felt good and she was smiling. I was not even trying to process the sounds and sights. Then suddenly I was. Perhaps it was the movement of the head of the blond lady, or the movement of her smiling lips saying something I did not process. Somehow, some force, was bringing me back at its pace. I felt an incredible, relaxed peacefulness just lying there accepting the situation without any thoughts of how or why. Perhaps it was spiritual caused by the greater force, or perhaps it was physical caused by the renewed flow of blood; probably it was a combination. I slowly returned to life one sense at a time. I could feel, then see, then hear, then recognize that there was a lady was looking down at me, then that there was a smiling crowd standing behind her. I had no idea what happened or, for that matter, no ideas at all. I was like a camera that records events without any interpretation. Thinking would come later: much later.

For me to have a second chance at life, the timing had to function as exact as the Astronomical clock in Prague has for over six centuries. Every tick, every minute, indeed every second, had to be effectively utilized. My only chance was to be in a cardiologist office: I was. No other place would have worked. If I had survived long enough to make it on the elevator down from the third floor of the cardiology department, overcoming the time requirements would have been almost impossible. The elevator takes at least three minutes for a round trip even if it is empty. If it was empty, then there would have been no one there to see me go down or hit the button to return to the cardiology department. If there had been other people on the elevator, there would have been confusion and other stops delaying my return past the crucial five minute mark for brain damage and probably the seven minute mark for survival. And that was my best chance. Any other place, all the time it would take to get me to the elevator would be added to the elevator time. For example, even if it was while I was walking to my car in the clinic's parking lot, brain damage would be a virtual certainty and survival almost impossible. While driving to the YMCA, a short three miles away, I would have crashed my car and maybe even caused injury or death to others. At the YMCA, the same questions would arise as did for the elevator at the clinic: how long before any one even saw me, recognized my problem, sought and found the proper equipment?

This brings up the second and third requirements: trained personnel with the proper equipment, which is a defibrillator. I suspect that most people's first reaction when I collapsed would be to try to revive me by speaking to me, followed by making me comfortable. These are the things I, and others, did years ago when one of our party collapsed in a restaurant in Pittsburgh. Fortunately he was not in cardiac arrest. I would not have been so fortunate. But, again, I was lucky as my cardiac arrest happened where the trained personnel with the proper equipment resided and who did not waste even a minute initiating appropriate corrective action.

While I have no direct knowledge of the events taking place after my cardiac arrest, a reasonable simulation would be: the narrow hallway on the third floor of the clinic where the incident occurred had a doctor, nurse, and technician walking quietly in rubber soled shoes while speaking in subdued voices; all would come to attention when the words "Code Blue" blared over the loud speaker and they would immediately rush to my aid. All medical professionals know that Code Blue is used when there is a cardiac arrest or respiratory arrest requiring Cardio Pulmonary Resuscitation (CPR) to restore breathing and circulation. Under Code Blue all medical personnel in a cardiac unit know success, or failure, will be quickly determined.

Urgency would be apparent everywhere, from the banging of coffee cups on desks, to the truncating of telephone calls, desk chairs scraping floors as they are pushed back, doors squeaking as they are yanked open, hurried voices making excuses over shoulders as personnel rush out of the other exam rooms looking at their watches. CPR teams would have the right-of-way in the narrow hallway as they rushed the cart with the defibrillator to the last exam room on the left: my room. Everyone would be aware that the clock had started ticking just before the Code Blue. Every second saved might help to save a life: the time for the technician and cardiologist to realize why I fell, the time to sound Code Blue, the time it took for the CPR team to process and react to the code, all counted against me.

When I taught time and motion study, we learned to break down everything into separate steps. For oral communications, the steps are the speaker thinks and then forms and speaks the words. At the speed of sound the words travel to the ear of the listener where it is transferred to his or her brain for interpretation. Listening occurs very rapidly, as the typical human can listen seven times faster than they can speak. The brain then sends a signal to the tongue and/or muscles for them to take action. All this happens quickly but not instantly: the tick tock continues.

The procedures call for personnel to hurry, but never rush, and never, ever, make any mistakes. Everyone in the hall would line the wall while the cart turns through the doorway into the last room on the left. All the relevant personnel had the training either on mannequins or each other, but almost no one had ever seen it applied to a real patient whose life hangs in the balance. My body will be their final exam. Like former students everywhere the first timers were reviewing their training.

The training to save lives would freeze all eyes onto the table while hearts hoped the body would show evidence of life: it did not. Clocks continued ticking as the defibrillator was brought into position. A defibrillator was used to deliver a therapeutic dose of electrical energy to the affected heart. The intent was to depolarize a critical mass of the heart muscle, terminate the arrhythmia and allow the body to reestablish its natural pacemaker in the sinoatrial node of the heart. Defibrillators transform electrical energy into the proper dose much like a transformer does for model trains. The electrical energy is delivered to the patient by means of two paddles. Applying the paddles requires a precise calibration of the amount of energy. Using too little might be ineffective and too much might simulate the effects of an electrocution. Even using the correct amount makes the entire body convulse. The wires are insulated so the operators do not get a shock. The first paddle is placed on the upper right side of the body opposite the heart and the other paddle placed on the lower left side. The slang for this procedure is "using the paddles" and has been popularized by television shows.

In my case, Dr. A's switching the defibrillator on would cause the electrical energy to race through the insulated wires and paddles into the body on the table. The body would convulse. All eyes in the room would be focused on the chest, every breath held as eyes strained to see the answer to the only question in the room: Was there movement? Suddenly the room would be full of sighs followed by every set of lips mouthing the same things: "Yes," and "Thank God." The heart of the body on the table had restarted. No longer was there a question of whether to call it "the" body or "his" body. It was Brent's body. Brent had been recalled to life. Was there brain damage?

I laid there in peaceful oblivion to what had just occurred. I looked at the blond lady rubbing my forehead and said the first words of my second life, "I want to sit up." The blond lady said, "You can't." For some indescribable reason I responded, "You don't understand, I have to." The blond lady looked over her right shoulder and a white coated man nodded his head up and down while saying, "Ok, but support his head." She put her right hand under my head and helped me raise it. It was tough and raising it all of five inches was enough to satisfy my urge. I slowly lowered it back to the table and never questioned why that was as far as I wanted to go.

Across town the conversation with my wife, Carol, did not resemble the relaxed nature of my first one in my second life. She was sitting at her desk in her office on the third floor, sometimes referred to as the executive floor, of a regional bank. As the Corporate Secretary she spends much of her days answering the telephone. On January 10th, she answered the telephone at 9:52 A.M. anticipating another call from a shareholder with problems. Instead the caller began, "This is a call from the cardiology department at the clinic. Your husband had a cardiac arrest but he has been stabilized and is being taken to the hospital." Carol's shock was complete. It is the call that no one ever wants or even thinks of getting unless your spouse has been deemed a high risk, which I had not been. She, like me, thought of me as the picture of good health. In some ways it might have been lucky that she went into shock since it produced a daze that may have prevented her from having her own cardiac arrest. We were also lucky that they had not called while I was transitioning (such a nice, mild word) from my first life through no life to my second life. Carol, after struggling to stand, wandered out into the hallway. She was confused and having trouble internalizing the call. Her mind was racing. Had her husband just had a cardiac arrest? She had just left him and he looked fine. Her father had died of an aneurysm at age sixty-two but he was overweight and did not exercise. Her older brother died in 2007 of a heart attack at age 58. She remembers thinking that I was sixty three but not that overweight and I exercised. In fact when she had last seen me, several hours ago, I was dressed for the gym. She staggered into the office next to hers, Debbie's office.

"My God, what is wrong," Debbie asked looking up from the work on her desk that immediately became irrelevant. Carol's face said it all. Debbie reacted quickly. She pushed back her chair, ran around her desk past her visitor's chair and wrapped her arms around Carol, saying, "What happened?" "The clinic just called and my husband had cardiac arrest," stammered Carol. Her demeanor made it obvious that she was incapable of making any decisions. Debbie, experienced from her first husband's death from cancer, gathered Carol's purse and half carried her to the garage, drove her to the hospital and helped her find me.

My ride to the hospital was less stressful, at least for me. My ride began when the gurney in the little room on the left started moving. I never thought of questioning why or where we were going. We were just moving. My view was looking up at the many faces whizzing by all silently looking down at me. We rolled down the beige hallway that I had walked down less than an hour ago. I read the overhead signs. As we turned left and approached the elevator, everybody stood aside. We caused a silence everywhere we went. People stood back and gave us room. The faces of the men and women in hospital attire reflected fear as they peered down at me as we passed. Visitors gasped while staring. My eyes saw and my ears heard the events but my mind was not processing them beyond noting that something about me was scaring everybody. Everything was surreal. I saw everything; I saw nothing. In a way it was like watching a silent movie in black and white. When the elevator doors opened, I heard gasping and shuffling. White coats hustled by me as they exited quickly. Others simply froze until told to disembark. I didn't try to talk but I thought, yes, it's me, Brent. I was not aware of being cold, or hot, or for that matter, being much of anything. No one else was on our elevator as it slowly descended past the second and first floors to the below ground floor. All this time would have counted against me if I had been in the elevator when my heart stopped. We took an underground tunnel under the street to the hospital. My clearest recollection of this, my first trip of my second life, is of ceilings; different substances, slightly different colors, most of them were sound proofing panels of a composite substance with little holes in neat rows and columns. They were all spotless, except for the stains on the ceiling in the tunnel.

This gurney ride again illustrated my defying the odds. I was lucky to have that gurney ride. Once my heart stopped, the alternative way to exit the clinic was gruesome. But even more than that, the underground tunnel to the hospital was only available in one of the 44 buildings of the clinic: the one I was in. My luck continued with the hospital at the other end of the tunnel, where the complete name for the department of the hospital was Emergency and Trauma Department. There is not another trauma unit within hundreds of miles. And I needed a trauma unit. "Trauma" means they are capable of handling even the most critical of problems, like heart problems.

During my gurney ride, Debbie was helping Carol find her way to the Emergency and Trauma Department. Carol found me behind a curtain still on my gurney. Her face conveyed her shock and fear as she hesitantly walked over to my side. I was still oblivious to my situation and almost everything else except, and it was a huge exception, I was pleased to see Carol. If it was possible for me to relax any more than I already was, I did at the sight of her. My mind did not process why she was with me. I can only guess at how difficult that must have been for her and even years later it is too painful to discuss. My awareness was limited to Carol when the emergency room doctor pulled back the curtain while saying, "We want to do an angiogram." I said, "No, I don't want it." Several times over the years I had vetoed cardiologist recommendations for this procedure since I was afraid of having a tube, that contains a tiny camera, inserted into my leg and threaded into my heart. This time Carol wisely said, "Do it, doctor."

An "angiogram" is a procedure for an x-ray test that uses a dye and a camera (fluoroscopy) to take pictures of the blood flow in an artery or vein (WebMD). The procedure is very accurate and the risk of major complications during this procedure, which may include a stroke or death, are rare (Mayo Clinic). The procedure is to insert a tube, called a catheter, into a blood vessel, frequently in a leg, and guide it towards the patient's heart. A micro camera is inserted into the heart through the catheter, enabling the physician to view the photos to determine where, if any, the blockage is located.. The procedure permits physicians to make relatively accurate assessment of the location of the blockage, as well as the amount of the blockage. Once the blockage is identified, the physician may use the catheter tube to perform an "angioplasty" to:

--insert a small balloon through the catheter into the arteries to hold them open by pressing the plaque against the artery walls, or

--grind (rotablation), shave (atherectomy) or cutting (cutting balloon) the plague, or most likely,

--insert a stent through the catheter into the inside of the artery to prevent the artery from becoming completely blocked. A stent is a tiny tube like structure, open at both ends, made of a material that will withstand pressure so it will maintain its shape and permit the blood to flow uninhibited. Some stents require the future use of drugs, such as blood thinners, and others do not.

Some things that seem conceptually so scary are, in reality, no big deal. The angiogram is nowhere near as bad as my fear of it. Perhaps it is the drugs. I am admitted to the hospital and wheeled up to my room where the first day of my second life will end.

I so defied the odds at every step of the way that I still can't believe we are talking about me. The odds of a "negative" experience during the exercise stress test have been estimate to have a probability of 0.0004, or one person in every 25,000 (ncbi.nim.nih.gov) and the odds of a "serious" negative result is one person in 100,000, or a percentage of 0.00001. The odds of surviving cardiac arrest were approximately three in 100, or 0.03. The probability of having my heart stop during an exercise stress test and then surviving a cardiac arrest becomes almost microscopic with an approximation being 0.0000003, or 3 in a million. That means that 999,997 out of every 1,000,000 who take a stress test would not have the same experience, and even fewer would not have brain damage. The number available to tell the story grows even smaller. And my defying the odds was just beginning. But the only thing that mattered was that my one heart would have the opportunity to support two lives!

CHAPTER 4. THURSDAY, JANUARY 11: HOW MUCH TROUBLE AM I IN?

"I have some bad news; your heart is in too bad a condition for you to be a candidate for a stent," one of the three men in white coats announced as they marched into my room. I did not understand him. Oh, I heard the words, and I knew what each of them individually meant, but I had no idea what the sentence meant. It was just a bunch of sounds. Whether it was the tone of the sounds or the frowns on the faces or the speaker that created a threatening feeling: I knew I had to focus. Who were these men in white coats? I looked around. Where was I? Nothing looked right. The walls were not yellow so this was not my bedroom. Where was I? Carol was there although I had just opened my eyes so we had not yet spoken. Why is this white coat talking to me? What is this about a stent? I tried to raise my right hand to my mouth, as I do when I am nervous, but it wouldn't come. Why not? I looked down and there were tubes sticking out of me. It appeared I was in a hospital room. Why? What happened? So many thoughts started running through my mind. I turned my head slightly to the right to look at the voice and said, "What?"

The voice came from a white coat, or actually the tallest of the three men wearing white coats, although their height was difficult to judge while I was lying on my back. He had thinning white hair and a serious, no nonsense look that, as strange as it may seem, also contained a comforting, friendly expression which softened his words of, "Good morning. I am Dr. W. a cardiac surgeon. Your angiogram, which is where we inserted a tube into your leg and threaded it up to your heart with a camera at the tip, enabled us to see into your heart. We hoped to be able to insert a stent but the angiogram showed the blockage in your arteries is 80%, 90% and 100%. Your heart is in too bad a condition for you to be a candidate for a stent."

I tried, unsuccessfully, to sit up a little straighter. The seriousness of his words was coming through, although the meaning had yet to become clear. My mind jerked to attention. He is a cardiac surgeon. Cardiac means related to the heart. Surgeons perform surgeries. Why was he visiting me? His other introductory words were lost on me. Apparently my face showed my confusion. His expression indicated I was in trouble. He said, "Your heart stopped." This is the first time I had heard this. Did it really stop? Stunned I blurted out, "Did I have a heart attack?"

The shortest of the three white coats stepped forth. I recognized him as the cardiologist from my stress test. I remembered him saying the test would be completed after the patient, me, had passed the six minute mark for recovering, and then his saying to the technician, "It has been five and a half minutes so you can start taking the electrodes off." I remembered I was telling him about my exercise program. That was the end of my memories. This morning he said, "Just before six minutes your heart stopped." Now I remembered how hard it had been to hold my breath while the trainee tech asked for directions on running the machine, so I asked him "How could I have passed the test if I had a heart attack during it?"

"You did not pass the test. Your heart stopped at the five and a half minute mark for recovery. We are going to use you in our training to teach folks that the test is not over until the full six minute mark," he said with a half-smile.

Listening to him was surreal in every way. My heart had stopped. He was telling me that I had not passed the test which didn't add up. I was wired during the entire time so there must have been some indications that the test should have been stopped. What good is a test if the patient dies before being told he failed? His nervousness and talking about a teaching moment told me something wasn't right. But I had to stay focused on the present and deal with him later, so I asked, "If I did not have a heart attack, what did I have?" "Your heart just stopped. It was out of rhythm," he answered.

Later I would learn that any disruption of the flow of blood to the heart may cause "angina." Symptoms of angina are frequently noticeable; such as pressure, tightness, aching, or pain in the chest, neck, back, arm or jaw. When a coronary artery is completely blocked the flow of blood to part of your heart would stop. That part of your heart muscles dies. This is called a "heart attack." The part that dies never returns to life. No part dies when the heart is out of rhythm. I asked him, "What caused my heart to stop?"

"Lack of potassium'" he replied. "Yours was below the standard."

"Lack of potassium," I repeated; my surprise being evident. "My heart stopped because of a lack of potassium?" Does he really believe this? Something isn't right. I have never had a potassium problem, including the recent blood work when my primary care physician shook my hand and congratulated me on the results. (Subsequently, a different cardiologist would confirm that low potassium was the effect, not the cause, of my heart stopping). At the time a couple of things were clear: I very much wanted to live, and pursuing this any further, at this time, would not help me live. So I asked Dr. W., the cardiac surgeon, "Did you say I had an angiogram?"

Dr. W. replied, "Yes and your coronary arteries are too blocked for us to be able to use a stent to reopen them."

What are my alternatives?"

Dr. W. explained that there were several ways to deal with coronary artery blockage. The choice depended on the extent of the blockage. When the blockage was not very great, a change in diet or exercise may be sufficient. At this time, these were not appropriate for me. When the blockage was greater, medicines may be prescribed to improve blood flow, lower blood pressure, or regulate heart rates. This was not available to me. When the blockage was even greater yet, the surgeon may perform an angioplasty to insert a small balloon through a catheter into the inside of arteries to press the plaque against the artery walls in order to hold the arteries open. The angiogram showed this was not available for me. A stent, could be inserted through a catheter into the inside of an artery to prevent the artery from becoming completely blocked. A stent is a tiny tube-like structure, open at both ends, made of a material that will withstand pressure so it will maintain its shape and permit the blood to flow uninhibited. This was not available to me.

My hopes increased each time the doctor mentioned another procedure available to physicians, only to be crushed as his words "not available" for me pushed me to slump a little lower in my hospital bed. I could feel my body tensing more each time he paused after saying "not available." Were there any choices left that might actually be available to me? I was in deep, deep trouble. What could he do?

He continued, "Your blockage of 80, 90 and 100% requires bypass surgery." Perhaps sensing from my expression that I felt like mine was a worst case, he continued, "There are some cases where the surrounding arteries or heart muscle are so weak that even by-pass surgery will not solve it. These folks are in serious trouble. You are not one of them. You are in overall good health."

This surgeon impressed me as a caring, straight forward, capable professional. This was my type of physician. Patients, like me, want to be told, in a polite way, exactly the problem and the alternatives for treatment. Thank goodness there were some things that could be done to help, and hopefully, cure me. I now knew I had had only one alternative, heart surgery, which I would learn is also called "by-pass" or "open heart" surgery. These discussions helped me mentally prepare for the only available alternative. Both the surgeon and I knew the choices were heart surgery and maybe live, or not. I appreciated being treated like a person rather than a case study. Mentioning that some people have problems worse than mine was a nice touch. "Are you going to schedule my surgery," I asked.

"Not so fast," he said as he turned to the third white coat. "This is Dr. C., a vascular surgeon. We agree that before your by-pass surgery we should run a test on your carotid arteries. Blockage, like yours, in coronary arteries frequently indicates there may also be blockage in your carotid arteries. You have two carotid arteries in your neck that carry blood to your brain; one on your right side and one on your left side. Plaque can build up in one, or both, arteries and reduce the flow of blood to your brain. Blockage in arteries reduces the area in which blood can flow, which raises blood pressure. For a partial blockage, aspirin or

Coumadin may be used to thin the blood to reduce blood pressure. More serious blockages may require surgery. We need to run an ultra sound test to determine if there is a blockage, and if so, how much is blocked.

Normally I will ask the alternatives to a test, but in this case it was painfully clear that it was necessary if I was going to survive. So I said, "Please schedule the test." Later in the same day a green suited woman pushed my wheel chair into a room tinted light gray without the benefit of windows, where a polite lady technician probably had no idea how terrifying she looked to me. She did her best to calm me. But it was hopeless. The technician politely asked me to climb into a dentist like chair where my neck was rubbed with a cool, thick jell as the tech said, "This will enable me to listen to the turbulence of the blood flow in your carotids." She sat on a stool on my right side, placed a stethoscope connected to the machine by a thin rubber tube, against the left side of my throat while saying, "This will measure the sound of the flow of blood in your carotids." I thought the sounds were loud but when she shifted to the right side of my neck, the sounds were scarily loud, with my best description being that it sounded like two whales mating where one was unwilling. My question, "How does it sound to you?" was answered with, "Please be quiet during the exam." My voice stayed quiet but my mind raced to interpret the sounds. Was a loud gurgling sound a good or bad sign? I searched my memory back 44 years to my fluid mechanics course for a hint. OK, decreasing the size of the pipe increases the pressure of the fluid, like squeezing a straw while trying to drink through it. Increasing the pressure increases the turbulence as the fluid enters the smaller area, so the louder the sounds, the smaller the passage area and the greater the blockage in the artery. I didn't like that opinion, so I tried to "read" the demeanor of the technician, but could not turn my head to see her. My perspiration increased until by the end of the test I was soaked. The technician deftly deflected my questions and I was wheeled back to my room.

In the afternoon, the cardiac and vascular surgeons burst into my room while saying, "There is bad news and good news. The bad news is your right carotid is either completely, or almost completely, blocked. The good news is that your left carotid is working fine." I remembered my friend F.X.O., leaning his six feet five frame over the small table in the converted stage coach stop called Buckley's Tavern, and saying in the no nonsense manner of a former Marine captain, "carotid arteries are important but they are not tested during routine annual physicals. If one is blocked your body can make adjustments. If they both are blocked: you die---quickly." Remembering this, I asked the vascular surgeon, "How can I function? How does the right side of my head receive blood if the right carotid is completely blocked?"

He replied, "Each carotid artery feeds a system of capillaries, which feed the cells in the brain. When one is blocked, our bodies adjust automatically to redirect the blood from the unclogged one to all over the brain. This is necessary as the brain can only survive for a few minutes without a blood supply since it does not store any blood." Only later would I wonder why my plaque had built up so much more in my right side than my left side, when both carotids were supplied by the same heart. My body had created a way to feed the right side of my brain with blood from the left carotid, but did it receive the same amount as the left side? The right side of my brain was the so called "emotional" side: was it receiving less blood? Did the lack of blood flow up the right side of my neck somehow affect the balance between the "emotional" right side and the "analytical" left side of my brain? Could my capillaries supply sufficient blood to balance both sides?

"What are my options?" I asked, to which he replied, "Normally the choices would be to either have surgery or just let you live with one functioning carotid, but if you did then it would be instantly fatal if the other one became blocked. But you don't have that choice, since without the surgery, called a carotid endarterectomy, there is a high risk of a stroke during heart surgery. Our surgery will consist of our cutting into your carotid and cleaning the plaque out with a drill like tool. The surgery takes between one and a half and two and a half hours."

I dread losing control under a general anesthetic. I try to justify it by thinking if cognizant, I will have the last chance to stop a problem. I know this is a rationalization as there undoubtedly would be nothing I could do during surgery, but it makes me feel better, so I said, "I don't want to go under twice. Can we do both surgeries at once?"

Both the doctors smiled: clearly they have heard this before. Dr. W. patiently explained that, "The risk of a stroke is greatly increased if the surgeries are performed simultaneously. If the heart surgery is done first, the potential blood pressure spike during the surgery might break some of the plaque in the carotid loose. There is a substantial chance that the loose plaque will travel through arteries and block the flow of blood to some part of your body. This blockage is called a stroke and it will be permanent. You may, or may not, lose part of your ability to think. You will certainly lose some mobility. We recommend that we do the carotid surgery before the bypass surgery. What would you like to do?"

What I would "like' to do is go home and forget the last two days. But I do appreciate being asked. I now believed that I was in serious trouble and the only way to live was to trust the experts. I asked, "What is the risk of death in a carotid surgery?"

"Virtually none for you as your overall good health is very much in your favor."

My thoughts were if my health is so good, what am I doing here? However, I really did appreciate the discussion and saw no reason to wait, so I said, "How soon can you schedule it?"

"Tomorrow, Friday," the vascular surgeon said. "That is as long as you don't have any more emergencies through the night. Before surgery any medical condition that increases the risk of strokes, such as high blood pressure or heart disease, needs to be controlled."

He got my attention. I was in such bad shape that I might not even be healthy enough for life saving surgery. I was afraid to ask my chances if surgery was not an option. Simply put: I must make it through the night without problems. I believed if I qualified for carotid surgery, I would survive it. I was not so certain about a stroke. If I survived intact, then I faced the more serious heart surgery. I tried to fully understand my chances of surviving, but doubted that I was successful. It was impossible for me to think of my fate beyond the two surgeries. My father used to say "A problem is only a problem until you identify a path to a solution. Then it is a process." I vowed to be as active a participant as I could.

My first step was to do all that I could to get ready for tomorrow's surgery. I knew movements increased blood pressure, so I decided to remain still all night and not move at all. My second day of my second life ended with my wondering if I will qualify for a surgery that yesterday I did not know I needed. I had learned through the three years and three months of helping my first wife, Anne, unsuccessfully battle cancer that it was only hopeless when the medical professionals ran out of procedures. When there was a medical procedure available, there was hope. Certainly it was a blow to learn I had heart problems, and another blow that they were so bad that I did not qualify for a stent.

One of my strengths has been dealing with what is real. As a lawyer, I had learned to first deal with the crisis and save trying to later determining the cause and then how to avoid a repeat. Thinking beyond the next procedure would distract my efforts from where they would be most constructive, so I focused on what I could do to make my surgery tomorrow a success. I viewed my role as a teammate to being part physical, which I dealt with by not moving, but mostly mental, for which I hoped, prayed and created a determination to not accept any outcome except success. I believe our thoughts can have an impact on our bodies, so my focus was on trying to send the message throughout my body that I, we, were going to do whatever it took to live and that we were in for the entire fight. I just hoped that I was strong enough to win with the help of the life creating force. I might have not known what really bad news meant when I woke this morning, but I not only knew by night but I also knew that it could get worse before morning if I moved too much. I straightened my arms and practiced the deep breathing that I had found so beneficial in yoga while I lay awake for most of the night with thoughts of how important life was to me.

CHAPTER 5. FRIDAY, JANUARY 12:
A PAIN IN THE NECK

My eyes flew open, my head jerked forward and my heart raced, but my world slowed down when I realized that I was alive at 6 A.M. on January 12th. This was Friday, the day of my carotid surgery. I quickly remembered the surgeon saying, "If you still qualify" and breathed a sigh of relief believing that I did. What a way to qualify: to not have another crisis in my heart. I dread surgeries but I love life, so here I was rejoicing. I had tried to stay awake all night after the surgeon said he would perform surgery if, and it was a big if, I did not do anything during the night to disqualify me. The only idea I had to continue to be "qualified" was to not move any muscle. Apparently I am very experienced at not moving as Carol was always amazed when I fell asleep in my recliner while holding a half full glass of red wine and would wake up without having spilled a drop. On this night I also was afraid that any time my eyes shut might be their last time. My body was still: my mind was not.

Dr. C., my white-coated vascular surgeon, entered and smiling asked, "Are you ready for your surgery? Our surgery is called an endarterectomy. We will make an insertion just under your jaw line, into your right carotid artery, and clean out the plague buildup. It takes between one and a half to two and a half hours."

It would be unfair to say that I was thrilled, but fair to say relieved and a little proud that I had done my part. I was surprised that I had a carotid problem, although to be truthful, if asked, I doubt that I had ever thought much about it either way. It is amazing how fast I learned something after it became a key to my continued living. After this was corrected, I vowed to learn how to prevent this situation from recurring. Maybe it was the drugs, or maybe I just didn't like the answer, that caused me to say, "Tell me again why we are not doing both the carotid and heart surgeries at the same time?" My fear of losing control was somewhat affirmed when, in law school, we studied a doctrine called the "last clear chance," which is applied to incidents where one person initiates something, like an automobile collision, the law asks who had the last clear chance to avoid it. I used this doctrine to justify my dislike of general anesthesia, although even I laughed at my thoughts that there was some way I could use my "last clear chance" during surgery.

"Having both surgeries together greatly increases the risk of a stroke," he said. "Because the changes in blood pressure necessary for heart surgery could cause some of the plaque built up in your carotid to break free and travel through your body causing a stroke."

I would later learn that a stroke occurs when the blood flow is cut off from part of the brain. Unlike most parts of our bodies, brains do not store any blood so any disruption in the flow immediately causes problems. There are two basic types of strokes: a hemorrhagic, where there is bleeding within the brain caused by a bursting blood vessel, and Ischemic, where there is a blockage of blood flow in an artery leading to the neck or brain (the National Institute of Neurological Disorders and Stroke (nind.nih.gov)). In the U.S., Ischemic, or blocked blood vessels, are responsible for about 80% of the approximately 800,000 strokes a year, making it the leading cause of serious adult disabilities. Strokes can also be fatal as about 150,000 people a year, or one every four minutes, die from strokes, making it the fourth leading cause of death. High blood pressure, high cholesterol and smoking are the major cause of strokes, and it is estimated that 49% of Americans have at least one of these conditions (Center for Disease Control and Prevention). Ischemic strokes are caused when fatty deposits, called "plaque," form in the arteries and by narrowing the interior width, reduce the space available for blood flow causing a condition called "atherosclerosis." The heart strains as it tries to push blood through the reduced space in the arteries. As the plaque continues to reduce the space even the increased strain on the heart can become insufficient to provide the needed blood to the body, which can cause a heart attack, stroke, or both, resulting in disability or death. Plaque tends to build up more in persons who lack physical activity, have an unhealthy diet or smoke, making them high risks. Hemorrhagic strokes are caused when chronic hyper tension of an aneurysm causes a blood vessel to burst. Although the risk of strokes increases with age, it is not limited to older persons as in 2009, 34% of the people hospitalized for strokes were under 65. Some persons with heart problems may appear to be "symptom free," so it is wise to consult a vascular physician to learn the various ways atherosclerosis may be detected.

My vascular surgeon had utilized an ultra sound test to screen for blockage. This non-intrusive test, meaning it did not permeate my skin, had felt strange but did not hurt. I wondered if I should have known that I had a carotid blockage. I am not certain whether I was symptom free since my tiring so quickly during exercise had been, in retrospect, a symptom of something. People can function with reduced flow in a carotid artery. When the accumulation is greater than 60% surgery may be used to cut the risk of a stroke in half for at least the next five years. Learning that the causes of the accumulation of plaque in arteries, such as lack of exercise, an unhealthy diet and smoking, were similar to those that caused fat to be accumulated on the outside of human bodies, I came to think of it as being "fat on my insides." This was quite a revelation as it indicated to me that just because I might not be overweight did not mean that I did not have a problem with fat, which might also indicate that some folks who eat all the wrong things but do not seem to have an external problem with fat may have an internal one that someday could be problematic. The National Institute of Neurological Disorders and Strokes provides a list of potential symptoms for carotid problems, many of which can occur simultaneously:

1. Strength, as with sudden numbness, weakness or paralysis in the face, legs, arms especially on one side of the body;

2. Sensation, as with sudden severe headaches which may last a few moments and then disappear;

3. Sight, as with trouble seeing with one or both eyes;

4. Speech, as with confusion talking or understanding speech; and slurred speech.

5. Steadiness, particularly if it occurs suddenly in walking, balancing or coordination.

I had not noticed having problems with any of these, but my wife reminded me that I did have sudden severe headaches that last a few moments. I had not experienced any sudden numbness, trouble seeing, talking or balance. As my right carotid was blocked, it was apparent that I must have missed a symptom. I sought a shorthand way to remember these five symptoms and decided that anything that originated above my neck might be a symptom.

On this Friday morning, while lying in my hospital bed, I acknowledged that my only warning about the risks of a clogged carotid artery had been one evening in the former stage coach stop, Buckley's Tavern, when my friend FXO, leaned his full six feet five inch frame a crossed the narrow table and, up close and personal, said in the voice of the Marine Captain he used to be, "If both of them are clogged, you die: quickly." Never again did I ever question the importance of carotid arteries, so I was not totally surprised when the vascular surgeon said there was a high risk of a stroke without first having the carotid surgery. I was suspicious of the low risk the surgeon gave for the surgery. I later learned that the Cleveland Clinic had estimated the risks of a stroke during carotid surgery as 1.7%, or a little less than two in a hundred, and the risk of death as 0.5%, or one person in two hundred. I was glad that if I needed a carotid surgery, they had determined it prior to my assuming the risks of a stroke during heart surgery. They had done their job. Now it was my turn. I visualized the process, as I always do as part of my "willing" the optimal result. Truthfully, I am not certain if my efforts help, but I know they won't hurt and they help me to relax. Ultimately, I know I must trust the surgeon. I tell myself that all those cases of malpractice we studied in law school were the exceptions, which is why we studied them. I was aware that my being an exception to the 97% who do not survive their heart stopping was responsible for my even being here, but now that the statistics were in my favor I wanted to just be average.

Fortunately, I did not have much time to wait. Normally, given time, I need to create a distraction so my mind will not focus on any negative things. I have never been a good at just waiting. Left alone, part of my brain will start to think negatively, while another part will argue that thinking negative is foolish. If the result is positive, there was no need to worry. If it turns out to be negative, worry about it then. The longer the wait, the more my emotional, or stress generating, side emerges. Waiting was always like this for me. One time while waiting for outpatient surgery my blood pressure spiked so much that the surgeon would not operate until it returned to normal. I was lying on an operating table in one of those gowns made for midgets. The anesthetic was supposed to relax me: wrong. I visualized the scalpel in the surgeon's hand slicing through my skin. The surgeon said "relax." My thought was that I'll relax when you put down the knife. Deep breaths were not much help while lying in that position. Finally, visualizing the faces of my children worked as it had when a dermatologist found a cancerous growth on my back and said he would run tests to determine the exact size and perform the surgery in two weeks. I said, "Have you done this type of procedure before?" Many times," he said smiling. "But with the proper test I might be able to cut out a smaller amount of flesh and still get it all." I responded, "I trust you. I will self destruct if I have to walk around for two weeks knowing I have a cancerous growth on my back. I am not getting off this table until you operate." The doctor gave a questioning look to Carol while asking, "He is serious?"

Carol never blinked when saying, "He is very serious." The doctor got the message and turned to me saying "lie still," while saying to his nurse, "Prep him. I only have one more patient for the day and I will see her in the other examination room. Then I'll operate." I did, she did, and he did. Ironically, and tragically, two weeks later, the time he initially wanted to operate, I returned for my post surgical check up and was stunned when I saw the doctor: both of his arms were in casts from his hands to his shoulders and were propped away from his body by metal rods connected to a special belt around his waist. He had no use of his hands. Suddenly my problem seemed insignificant. This dermatologist, who appeared to be in his early thirties, said, "While standing on a ladder at home, I lost my balance and fell backwards through a plate glass window. The glass cut the arteries in both my arms. The prognosis for my recovery is uncertain. In the meantime, my wife has to do everything for me: She dresses, feeds and even shaves me." I was so upset about his problems that it was days later before I realized had I not insisted on the earlier surgery, the day of my check up would have been the day of my surgery. Sometimes I think of the dermatologist as an example of how quickly an unexpected event can change our lives.

On this Friday, January 12th, to calm my nerves while the time for my surgery kept slipping, I found that breathing deeply and picturing the faces of my children did help, at least enough so I could almost sit still. I took some comfort from thinking that I was being bumped because my condition was not as serious as other patients. One result of having been involved in numerous medical situations was learning that for every rule there were exceptions; such as the time an orthopedic surgeon had shared his frustrations at being in charge of scheduling the surgical rooms with the words, "Frequently surgeries would be backed up not because of an emergency but because a surgeon, or patient, was late."

Finally the orderlies arrived. Funny, isn't it that after wishing for something, when it occurs you sometimes wished that it hadn't? A slight push and my gurney and I began our journey. Thank goodness Carol walked next to me. This can be a lonely journey. I was given a drug strong enough to calm me down but not strong enough to make me unconscious. I needed distractions but I was unable to have a conversation. I felt guilty putting that burden on Carol. I remembered the times I had been the one walking besides the gurney searching for something to say to make the patient more comfortable: something interesting, something personal as national news is of no interest to one that may be facing their maker; something meaningful and not trivial. I never found such a topic. Not when I was holding the hand, hoping not for the last time, of Carol before her surgery for breast cancer, my first wife Anne for her surgeries for breast and then liver cancers, and my sister Jill for vaginal cancer. Being the last person standing next to a love one's gurney is a great privilege and a solemn duty. A privilege to offer comfort, and a duty to show courage and support so they can pass through the swinging doors knowing they are loved. To my chagrin, I was aware that I never seemed to have found the words of comfort I was searching for. Now that I was on the gurney, I realized the topic was irrelevant: what was relevant was just being there.

Carol was not permitted into the pre-surgical room where I only paused before being pushed through the swinging doors into the operating room. It might have been my nerves, but the banging of my gurney against the swinging doors seemed like a cannon. The operating room was much larger than I expected. Its walls were lined by dark, ominous looking machines. I wondered why they were stored in here until reality hit: they weren't being stored; they were in case something went wrong during my surgery. The figures in gowns reminded me of the ones in horror films as they looked down at me over their white masks, while holding their hands in the typical pre-surgical position. My body started tingling from the emotions screaming "It's not too late. Get out of here," which was overwhelming my analytical side. A voice broke the quiet by saying, "Move him onto the center table." Nervous to fight my urge to run, I started to move myself onto the table before a no nonsense voice said, "No, we will move you." Once on the table, a mask was placed over my nose and mouth. I was not given any instructions, but I needed to be an active participant, so I needed to make my own: but how? Ah ha, I thought, as my mind jumped back over 50 years to when I was having my tonsils taken out and the surgeon told me to count down from 100. I had a vivid image of his laughing when I asked what to do when I reached one.

This time I did not ask. I just started doing my part: 100, 99...91, nothingness. The procedure that had caused my day to start with my eyes wide open and my heart and mind racing, now forced my eyes to peacefully shut and my heart to slow. My mind would was a different story. My body entered the land of nothingness comforted by my belief that the anesthetics might eliminate my conscious memories of this time, my strong self conscious desire to fight to live might make a difference.

CHAPTER 6. SATURDAY, JANUARY 13: HOW TO SPEND MY LAST DAY ALIVE?

"How to spend what may be my last day alive," was a question I had never considered. That is, not before this Saturday, January 13th. As my grogginess of another night in a hospital began to fade, my memories returned. I had survived my carotid surgery. The relief on Carol's face was a powerful incentive to affirm my commitment to continue my fight to live. If other things happened last night, they were not important enough to remember. I had won the right to live another day: today. How would I know if I had a stroke? I looked through all the connecting tubes and my room looked the same. I seemed to be able to move my arms (at least a little), as well as my legs. No parts of me hurt and I was not experiencing any numbness. I didn't know what symptoms to look for and I did not want to scare or possibly put her in the position of having to tell me any bad news. If I couldn't handle a bad answer, I was better off not asking. Two white coats entered and the vascular surgeon said in an excited voice, "Congratulations, your carotid surgery was a success." As they continued toward my bed, he repeated, "Your surgery was a success."

This gave me the courage to blurt out, "Does that mean I did not have stroke?"

"Of course not," he said. "I told you the surgery would be successful, and it was. I cleaned out your right carotid, which was completely blocked. The surgery took longer than we expected but the result is what we hoped for."

Suddenly it was easier to breathe. I smiled; I think. My body sank down into the bed. Now that the full flow of blood to my brain was restored, would I think or feel any differently? The taller white-coat, the cardiac surgeon, Dr. W., stepped forward and said, "We are cleared for your bypass surgery. Assuming you still qualify, would you rather I perform the surgery tomorrow or Monday?"

Whoa, not so fast. I just survived major surgery. How can I answer that question? I stammered, "Tomorrow is Sunday--- Can you perform surgery on a Sunday?"

He smiled as he said, "I actually prefer performing surgery on a Sunday as we will be the only one scheduled, so we can take as long as we want."

Of course he knew tomorrow was Sunday. I just needed some time to process his question, so to buy time I asked, "Can you get a full support team together on Sunday?"

While he was answering with perplexed look on his face, "Of course," my desperate search for some standard to use to evaluate his question led to my question: what possible standard could there be to determine whether to have heart surgery tomorrow or the next day? Getting a second opinion would be impossible, so what would I gain by waiting? I liked the idea of his not being rushed. If I am not going to survive the surgery, having it on Monday would give me another day to live. I would pick Monday if I could reach out to my children on Sunday, but I couldn't. Until surgery, I will be lying in Intensive Care with no telephone, no internet, no note pads, and no way to share with my family what might be my last thoughts. I decided that if I survived, I would do a better job of sharing my feelings with them. If I am going to survive, having it Monday would only increase my worrying time. I asked Carol what she thought. To her great credit her answer was "It is up to you."

"Tell me again my chances of survival," I asked the surgeon.

He said, "Your chances are very high. Based on your age and health, your chances are almost 100%." Now those words were almost reassuring. The "almost" was because a voice kept saying that if I was in such great health, what was I doing here? Almost did not feel too comforting when it involved life or death. Besides starting with my heart stopping, I had defied the odds so much that I no longer thought they applied to me. I took comfort, again, in my father's saying that a situation was only a problem until you took some action to correct it, and then it was a plan, so I said to Dr. W., "Sunday it is."

"Then I'll see you tomorrow morning, if you qualify," he said.

"Wait a minute," I stammered. "There is a chance I might not qualify for life saving heart surgery?"

"Yes. If your condition worsens we may not be able to perform the surgery."

I thought choosing the day to decide my fate would be the hardest part of my day: I was wrong. The hardest question was how should I spend what may be my last day alive? What were my choices? If I didn't survive the surgery, whatever I did today would make no difference, and if I did survive, the answer was the same! Wait a minute. That's not true! If I wake up after the surgery, then I will have a second chance at life. What can I do today to start to improve this second chance? Perhaps it would be a constructive use this day to review my life to see what I might wish to change?

I had suspected that I had more sources of stress than most people, since my drive for the unspecified goal of "perfection" made me a "stress generator." I had thought my propensity to generate stress was the secret to whatever successes I might have achieved, although I had wondered if one day the balance would shift from eustress, or good stress, to distress, or bad stress, and convert my greatest strength, my drive, into my greatest weakness. I felt the key to preventing the transition was to maintain "stress relievers," which were exercise and relaxing at home. I was somewhat in balance until 1981, which ironically coincides with the 20-25 years that the medical profession feels it takes for the effects of stress to be evident. I had a general understanding of some of the causes of stress, which years later were listed on Web.MD as:

-Death of a love one   -Increased financial obligations
-Divorce   -Moving
-Loss of a job   -Having a heavy work load
-Taking care of elderly or sick family member

Unfortunately, as will be discussed in the following pages, my life included illustrations of all of these and a few more.

In 1981, I had settled into my position as an attorney. My wife

Anne and our three children: Chad, Hollie and Grant, who were respectively, 8, 6 and 4, were happy with our lifestyle in Kingwood, Texas. Then I decided to take a chance to further my career by accepting a new job that required a "move" to Los Angeles. While looking for a house, I began spending Monday through Friday in L.A. and flying back to spend the weekends with my family. All our moving plans were put on hold when Anne, after finding a malignant lump in her breast, followed her oncologist recommendation and had a partial mastectomy followed by a brutal version of chemotherapy: she was hospitalized for one week every three months where every morning she was given an IV of sterilized tuberculosis to raise her temperature to the desired 103 degrees Fahrenheit. Since closely tracking the uneven rise was difficult for the staff, my role, besides comforting her, was to closely monitor the rise because at 107 degrees there was such a serious risk of brain damage that a team would rip off her sheets and throw ice water on her already shivering body. Seeing this once was enough, so I spent as many nights as possible in the hospital.

The stress I felt at not being able to prevent her from suffering defies words! I can, however, illustrate it by discussing the time my back went into such spasms that I had to roll off my temporary sleeping arrangements, on the cot at the foot of Anne's hospital bed, and take short, hunched over, half steps to the lobby, since Anne's hospital did not treat backs, before waiting out front for a taxi. I squinted at the sunlight, that I had not seen in days, while wondering "how all these people are going to work? Don't they know Anne is fighting cancer?" After the cab took me to another hospital for pills, I returned to Anne's bedside.

There was a time when the agony in Anne's gasp as a "doctor" erroneously punctured her lung, while performing a procedure, so overwhelmed me that I felt the heat rush to my head and my right arm automatically drew back to punch the face of the person who was hurting my wife. The doctor ran from the room with my words, "If you ever come near my wife again, I will break your face" bouncing off his back. We were both fortunate that my tending to Anne prevented my pursuing him down the hall. Later the head of his practice said, "After that doctor failed the qualifying test in Kentucky, we decided for diversity purposes to give him another chance." I never saw that doctor again.

Anne's parents, known as momma and poppa to my children,

were nice enough to fly to Houston and stay with my family while I worked in L.A. Later I realized that the shrinkage in my well stocked bar coincided with the increased bizarreness in momma's behavior, although it wasn't until years later that I learned that she used to say to my 6 year old daughter, "See this chain around my neck. I am going to tighten it a little more each day until I kill myself. I don't want to live."

Anne kept her good spirits but lost her hair, appetite and, sometimes, her mobility, but never her grace. She fought a quiet fight not wanting to upset the family by telling the children she had cancer. She spent her 40th birthday in the hospital eleven days before mine.

I had a "loss of a job" when I returned to Houston, which was now in a recession, to care for my family. After "increased financial obligations" caused problems, I accepted a position with a company best described in two words by a friend from Exxon: "I'm sorry." For a couple of years I entered an office where my legal and personal ethics were challenged. Subsequently the CEO went to jail. Based on my years of practicing law and having been successful in court as well as in mock trials at the world class training course for trial work, the National Institute of Trial Advocacy (NITA), I thought I was ready for the fifty cases I inherited: wrong! These were like cases rarely seen in corporate America. We had no documents or witnesses to support our questionable legal allegations. Simply put they should never have been filed, but would be easy victories if the other sides ever filed the appropriate motions. My twelve hour days of striving for the balance between maintaining my ethics while representing this client wore me down so much that one night I paused in my front door way: was I was coming from, or going to, work?

At home we had some good moments, such as playing soccer, basketball, swimming, and riding bikes over, and around, the rattle snakes crawling on the green belts. However, the stress of being a care giver interrupted every personal thought with, "How can you be thinking about yourself when Anne is in such trouble?" My mantra became, "You can do whatever is necessary to get through today, including, if necessary, standing on your head," although the endless sequence of "todays," slowly ground me down over the three year, three month period of Anne's cancer spreading to her back, where radiation stopped it, then to her liver, where surgery stopped it, and then everywhere. I will never forget the relief on her face as she left us at age 42. Watching the ghost like translucent, white cloud flow upwards out of her body changed my life: forever. Since our first date at 17, we had been inseparable.

I had lost my life partner! My time as a caregiver for my wife had ended but my role as a parent-caregiver for our children, at ages 8, 10 and 12, who had just lost their mother at about the same age that my father had lost his, continued. On a walk, I said to my children, "I have been watching you guys and I think you are doing ok." My daughter said, "We have been watching you, too, and you are doing ok too." I was surprised, and thrilled, at the caring and maturity of that conversation. The first housekeeper I hired had a 50% absent record; the second stole things; the third took my children with her while she cleaned a dentist office at night; there was no fourth: We were on our own!

Within four months of Anne's passing my new boss of one month laid off the entire law department, including me, except for the one attorney who had the company's secrets. In a way it was a relief. I had lost interest in doing litigation, which I had come to see as "recreating the past in the light most favorable to my client," as thoughts of the past kept reminding me of Anne's suffering.

We moved to a small town in Pennsylvania with the promise that I would succeed the diabetic VP who, on my first day of work, was in the cardiac ward of the hospital bragging about how he snuck cigarettes in the waiting room: within six months he was dead. The company then proved the axiom that "an oral promise is not worth the paper it is printed on," when it declined to honor our agreement. I knew my time there was ending when a senior manager of one of our facilities, a battle hardened retired colonel, self consciously wiped the tears from his eyes as he related that he knew telling me of the numerous, overwhelming, indisputable instances of sexual harassment by my boss would save his staff while costing him his job. I saved his job but not my own.

The first, and last, time I saw momma and poppa after Anne's death happened when I unexpectedly was home during a summer week day when, after driving hundreds of miles, they "stopped in." Poppa said, "Not a day goes by that I don't think that you killed my daughter, because if you had not advised Anne to have a partial mastectomy, she would have had a full one and be alive today." I was stunned! Saying, or thinking this, was so far outside my scope of understanding that all I could do was blurt out the truth, "I told her it was her life and her choice." As we bid them *adieu* I knew we would never see them again, and we never did. Later I realized blaming someone else a theme I had heard from him for over 25 years, and I wondered what plans they had for my children that my unexpectedly being home had spoiled.

Midnight on a Friday night that summer I received a call that the police were holding my 16 year old son for a violation of a curfew that prohibited anyone under 18 from being out after 9 P.M. The cleaned up version of what the policeman said was that the next time he would take my son to the detention center and let some big guy teach him the facts of life. I said, "Don't you think being raped is kind of a stiff penalty for a curfew violation," while thinking two things: this policeman is seriously unbalanced and we had to move.

I had recovered sufficiently from my grief that I was able to accept a position of Chief Employment Counsel with Hercules Incorporated in Wilmington, Delaware. Within a year I expanded my predecessors responsibilities of the legal aspects of 32 collective bargaining agreements to include all legal issues from recruitment-to-retirement for 26,000 employees worldwide. This hectic practice included being trial counsel while winning the largest contested case in the history of OSHA (in the World Trade Center) as well as several precedent setting cases on drug testing and age discrimination. Yet these stresses of these paled in comparison to those of being assigned to travel to every facility to reorganize them and eliminate 10,000 jobs. My stress reliever was my daily lunch time jogs along the Brandywine River, or early morning ones in the city of the day. On the road, there were many nights when I sat in lonely hotel bars with intertwining worries about how my children were doing at home alone and about the families of the employees whose jobs I had just eliminated. Was I that guy that my father had feared would someday arrive from corporate and eliminate his job? The only way I was able to continue to face myself each morning was to conclude that the CEO and VP of HR, both my age, who during this time both had heart attacks, had identified me as the "right" guy. I received some comfort from the operations people realizing that my unique education, experience and judgment provided a foundation for objective, business driven decisions, which was reinforced when, to be able to counsel the facilities whose solid fuel rockets had been used by

President Reagan to negotiate the end of the Cold War, I received a Top Secret security clearance which, at one point, enabled me to take charge of a black box that was to be used if the U.S. was attacked!

My family was functioning, although I never had the time to give my children the time they wanted, or deserved. When facing my 50th birthday, I faced the reality that I was in danger of not being able to finance my children's educations, or to be able to back away from the stresses before they put me on my back. A statistic from the American Trial lawyers Association (ATLA) haunted me: the life expectancy of a trail lawyer was 56!

To provide some direction to my life, I decided to write my first life plan. I was clueless how to start so I asked myself: what were my goals in life and how could I create a plan to achieve them? After living for so long from day-to-day crisis, which I came to call my "crisis *de jour*," I knew my general goal was to live a "happy, healthy life," but now, for the first time, I needed to be more specific. I saw that while increased finances would not guarantee happiness, without a large increase in income it would be impossible for me to finance my children's educations or my retirement.

I sought the assistance of a professional financial firm, who produced a very detailed financial plan that balanced returns with risks over a twenty year period. It was similar to my previous twenty year plan that had been exhausted in supporting my family through our turmoils and tragedies. I agreed with this type of plan for anyone who has at least a twenty year horizon. However, as my children were approaching college age and I retirement, this no longer included me. Unfortunately the only prudent strategies I could find for my new time horizon, five to seven years, focused on protecting, rather than creating, resources. But only protecting my now insufficient resources would guarantee failure. My only hope was to take chances that no prudent advisor could, or should, agree with. I like to think I reasoned (but probably "rationalized" is the better word) that none of us were born with any investment skills, so all of them were learned skills, and if someone else could learn them, then so could I. A word of caution: I do not recommend this approach. It was incredibly difficult and stressful. Every one of my days began, and ended, with the my trying to master the mysterious stock market. I spent the time in-between doing parenting things for my three children, running a household and and practicing law. Reducing sleep and recreational activities would have been insufficient if my children were not so great, my career having advanced to the point where I could reduce my research time, and the time being right for my greatly overweighting technology: I met my goals in five years.

My mother inadvertently demonstrated the stress of "taking care of an elderly family member," as well as the importance of acting promptly to deal with health issues. After her second husband, Charles, died of cancer, she lived alone in very rural Smith Mountain Lake, Virginia. My pushing her wheel chair into the cancer center of Wake Forest University opened my eyes to how desperate she had become, as well as her need for surgery. Subsequently her postponing her surgery forced a surgeon, on an emergency basis, to amputate her leg above the knee, where the prosthesis had to substitute for two joints. Besides frequent visits, I called her every morning.

One night, as I was sitting in my recliner in Delaware with my cat Muffie in my lap, I gave out. Being alone was no longer an alternative as Carol had moved to Santa Barbara for career advancement, Chad and Hollie were in San Diego, and Grant was in Honolulu. In January, 2001, I accepted an offer from a financial firm for a position in California after a six-week training period in New York, where every morning I had walked through the World Trade Center (WTC). When the terrorists blew it away on 9/11, they also blew away my job. While my loss was trivial compared to so many others, it hurt as did the resulting stock market crash that eliminated much of my retirement funds. Wars and depressions can have a devastating effect!

My stress reliever became my Delaware house until a branch cut a hole in the roof permitting water to create mold in the walls causing the insurance adjuster to declare my house not habitable and advising me to take what I needed to live for a "couple of weeks." As the time dragged on, I began to feel like my identity had been stolen: all my financial records, family heirlooms, furniture, clothes, art works, in short every physical object I identified with, and cared enough to accumulate over my lifetime, were being controlled by persons that would turn out to be thieves waiting for the right opportunity. After the damage was done, the the adjustor was fired, and the alleged "certified mold contractor" (since I had learned there is no such certification) left the state with his stolen booty, I hired a "friend" to solicit bids for rebuilding. Unfortunately, he "joined the crowd" by falsely listing himself as the lowest bidder.

It would become a costly mistake to trust him. Absent a place to live in Delaware, I spent most of my time in California until I learned the "friend" had told an electrician not to worry about installing safety devices by saying, "Don't worry, if the house burns down I won't tell him who did the work." After I returned, without telling him, I fired him after he did not show up at the job site for eleven days. A skilled carpenter subsequently refused the job, saying "The work your contractor has done is so bad that I do not want my name to be associated with it." Another carpenter insisted on first filming my "friend's" mistakes so he would not be blamed for the incompetence, such as the large ceiling fan in the family room that was only attached to wall board so that when turned on it would fall. The projected 90 day project took three years and not even including the insurance company's payments, my out-of-pocket costs were double the estimates for the entire project. An illustration of my stress was the time I chased a driver around my front lawn after he returned a pile of junk instead of my 53 inch surround sound television. There were times that I wished my house had burned down. At the beginning of this three-year period a friend had said, "Don't let this kill you, as it too shall end:" six months after it ended my heart stopped.

My review provided a perspective on the increases in stress that had begun at age sixteen when I realized I had to take responsibility for myself. At first most of the stresses were the positive eustress, which later became distress due to all things I cared about, but could not control, as a student, husband, parent, child of aging parents, bread winner and, sadly, widower. My expanded activities required that I trust others to manage but for which I kept trying to maintain responsibility.

I learned that unless I took care of myself, I would not be able to help my family, friends, community or country. Things can be replaced but the loss of principles, or people, cannot. I lost my battle with stress. But maybe, just maybe, not the war. As I had told my mother, "You have a lot of reasons to fight for life." Now it was my turn.

Unbeknownst to me at the time, this review of my life would be the beginning for developing "Managing Your (my) Rehabilitation Program WELL." (When used herein, capitalized and in quotation marks because of the alteration of the title of this book).

CHAPTER 7. SUNDAY, JANUARY 14TH: PREPARING FOR HEART SURGERY

My judgment day had arrived! Today, this Sunday, January 14, 2007, was it! Today will either be my last day, or the first day of "One Heart---Two Lives" having a chance to become a reality. Was I ready? I believed the surgeons answer of "yes" was the best alternative for my leaving Intensive Care. But was I emotionally ready? My review yesterday had helped, as it being a Sunday also did, but is anyone really ready? Isn't that why suicide is prohibited? In the end, doesn't it always come down to faith?

For me the debate was over. There would be no more waiting, planning or praying: today was it. Today a cardiac surgeon will try and correct the damage that I have done to the work of my creator. My spirit was ready for the fight. My heart will be first to know the outcome, followed quickly by my brain, organs, muscles, bones and finally after the anesthetic wears down, my consciousness. Tonight every part of me will enjoy the increase in the blood flow, or suffer from the restrictions of a stroke, or no longer function at all. Tonight I will either be better, worse, or gone, but definitely not the same.

I wished I hadn't put the surgeon in the position of having to save me and, given a chance, I would never, ever do it again. I wanted my full, independent life back. If I knew any way to have it besides heart surgery, I would do it in a New York minute. But there was no middle ground. Today I either get better, or worse. Death had become personal when my wife, Anne, passed. I knew it had caused me to think a little differently than others my age. The effects on my children had been significant and while I had done everything I knew how to do to help soften their loss, I also felt that a loved one should be missed.

I was scared and exhausted from not sleeping. Logical thinking was that I had to sleep, but whenever I dozed my head tilted to the left and my emotions jerked me awake. Stress was highliting the competition between the logical and emotional approaches emanating from my brain. As a broad generalization of an incredibly complex organ, the two main sections of the human brain are the left and right hemispheres. The left hemisphere, or the "left side," is associated more with originating logical, analytical or objective thoughts. The right hemisphere, or "right side," is associated with originating more intuitive, thoughtful or subjective thoughts. For illustrative purposes herein the "left" side of the brain will be used to represent logical, or analytical thinking, and the "right" side to represent more emotional thinking. The over simplification of the workings of the brain is intended to illustrate the difference between logical and emotional approaches that exist in everyone.

On this morning of heart surgery my "axons," which relay messages between the hemispheres in brains, were active. The subjective right side of my brain kept saying, "You are in the hands of a good surgeon who seems to know what he is doing." The objective left side, asked "Why do you think he is good? A confident bedside manner is not necessarily an indication of surgical competence."

The right side said, "But we don't have his surgical record, and even if we did, we wouldn't know how to evaluate it." The left side then asked, "Then why do you trust him?"

The right, "I guess it is because we have to: he is all we've got." The left side, "We should have gotten a second opinion."

The right side said, "How were we going to get a second opinion while lying in Intensive Care lucky to be breathing. Besides it has only been one day since the carotid artery on my side of the neck was re-opened to provide an increased blood flow directly to me." The left side, "Congratulations and I am glad to no longer have to share mine."

The right side, "Staying positive for the carotid surgery helped while we were under the anesthetic so I, we, can again help the surgeon by visualizing the surgery and willing our body to help. A couple of days ago we were a walking time bomb with less than a five percent chance of surviving. Beating these odds required the help of a force a lot greater than luck. Then, if we were even strong enough to qualify, we needed multiple surgeries. Now we only need one more surgery: but a huge one. If we wake up from this one, we can start recovery." The left side whispered, "If we haven't had a stroke."

The right side, "Time is short. The increase in blood makes me certain that I know the odds. I understand you may disagree, but I believe." The left side, "I believe belief is powerful, so I will stop arguing. We are in this together."

I jolted out of my grogginess. My head jerked upright. My eyes opened wide. My shoulder muscles tightened. My heart rate quickened. The countdown had begun. Immediately before surgeries, my focus shifts to my fear of anesthetics. It was a deep seated one that I first became aware of when I was in second grade. Before my eye surgery, I told the surgeon that I was afraid to be unconscious. The surgeon telling me that if I was awake I would be able to see directly into my mouth after they took my left eye out and laid it on the side of my face, at least stopped that fear for that surgery. What a lesson for surgeons that their words matter even to seven year olds. Unfortunately the surgeon's message was not complete as when I woke after surgery I could not see anything, not even any light! Was I blind? I learned that they had bandaged both my eyes shut so the muscles on my "good" eye, the right one, would not pull the left's muscles while they were healing. For the next week I could not see anybody: my parents, the nurses, the boy in the next bed, or anything; the looks on the faces of my parents, doctors or nurses, or the food being spooned into my mouth. My hands never let go of my new cast iron truck that was colorless until my parents told me it was red. All days became nights with different sounds and occasionally smells. My seven-year old mind wondered if I would I ever be able to see again. This may have been the beginning of my obsession with opening my eyes post surgery began, as well as knowing what to anticipate.

Unknown to me at the time there was another valuable lesson forming. When the voice of the boy in the next bed, whom I never saw, went home a day before my release, I told the doctor that I wished I was him. I vividly remember the doctor very gently replying that this boy had already had a series of surgeries, would be returning for another one and may never be cured from the pieces of steel in his eyes. It was a long time before I realized the lessons arising from my concern for the boy: watch what you wish for, stay focused on the results and do not get too discouraged or distracted by temporary discomforts. Unfortunately, I frequently forget this lesson.

After being told that I would be under for over eight hours, I changed my focus from the anesthetic to the surgery. I visualized the surgeon drawing a line down my chest before tracing it with his scalpel. Whoa, all I could visualize for the next step, that of his opening my ribs, was the crude way that I would crack and open a crab at Phillips Crab House. This was not good. I shifted my focus to the remarkable design of our bodies where the vital organs are protected by a strong set of ribs and I remembered a quote from, I believe, Albert Einstein, that has frequently provided comfort, "The more I study the body, the more I believe anything designed so magnificently could not have occurred by chance."

In my layman's terms, this time I anticipated that the balance was for the surgical team to ensure that I received sufficient anesthetic to slow my heart down so the surgeon could perform his surgery while my heart still pumped blood, although visualizing it pumping in my opened chest was tough. The surgeon had explained that in the event that it could not, the circulation of my blood would be assisted by an external pump. The pump, crudely referred to as a "blood pump," creates blood pressure by pushing the blood through narrower tubes and then returns it to the body for circulation. Sometimes the compression slightly changes the internal structure of the blood. This can lead to post surgical problems. I viewed my role as training my subconscious by visualizing my surgery without a pump as well as my waking up to find that I did not have a stroke during the surgery.

Facing this was one of the scariest things I had ever done. Facing it alone must be a desperate feeling. The orderly entered my room. It was time to begin my journey. Carol walked besides my gurney, as I am, for the second time in three days, wheeled down the hall to a door where the orderly said to Carol, "This is pre-op. You cannot go in." Carol kissed me, told me she loved me and before my eyes completely filled; my gurney and I were pushed into pre-op.

Normally the only comfort in a cold, stark pre-op room is the other patients. Today, this Sunday morning, there were none. The gurney driver parked me on the right side, halfway between the door I entered and the one on the right through which I will exit, and left. I was alone in this large, cool, sterile, empty room; realizing that certain things each of us must face alone; like entering and leaving this world. A nurse stepped out of the office in the far left corner and walked directly to me. She leaned forward and started with the expected question: Do you know the type of your surgery? I answered "open heart surgery." I had expected this question since we had read about why they asked it in law school: because it might prevent busy surgeons from performing the surgery scheduled for patient x on patient y. I was not surprised when other procedures meant to prevent mistakes, such as writing "this leg" on the leg intended for surgery, were not asked before heart surgery. But I was really stunned when the nurse leaned over the railing of my gurney and whispered," Have you ever had an out-of-body experience?"

Let me assure you that while I was lying in a gurney waiting for heart surgery, I was listening carefully. My problem was not the words: it was their meaning. Had I possibly misunderstood her? Did I hear her right? Did she really ask that? As I started searching for a response, my subconscious sprang into action. It was amazing. It was like my conscious mind had been frozen as a series of scenes flashed by in an instant. The first ones made me smile: Anne as a seventeen year old in her gown for the Snowball dance, our first morning as a married couple, waiting in the hallway for the birth of our first child, standing in the hospital next to Anne while holding each of our three children for the first time, our family standing by our first house and the effort to build our first family snowman. Then, without warning, the visuals started making me sad: very sad. Anne sitting in a hospital gown in a hospital bed in the oncology ward looking at me with tears running out of her eyes as the chemo made her sick. The scene flashed to her sitting in the back seat of our car on the way to Corpus Christi complaining about back pains that we would learn meant the cancer had spread to her back, then to my physically chasing the physician out of her hospital room after he had erroneously punctured her lung while inserting a medical apparatus, helplessly standing next to her as time-after-time a physician would say that the cancer had spread first to her back, then liver, then lungs and finally everywhere as her body ran out of energy. I was by her side when I saw the relief come over her unconscious body as the fog like substance, which I believe was her spirit, left her body traveling upward. At that moment something inside me changed: I just sagged.

The visuals continued to my telling my children that their mother had died, before flashing forward even faster through the next weeks with me in a trance-like state, as my friends J.G., George and Tina, were taking charge of the arrangements. I functioned in a zombie-like state; going through the motions of managing the litigation cases, home, children, dinner and sleep.

Weeks later a secretary in my office, who was helping to organize the pile of medical bills, invited me to follow her home after work so we could resolve some questions away from work. At her place something inside me broke. Without saying a word, she just stood up and led me into her bedroom. During my first intimate contact in over three years, I became aware that I was looking down at my back from a distance of a couple of inches. My spiritual self, for lack of a better designation, was slowly rising straight up towards the ceiling. I remember thinking that this is the first time I have ever seen my back without mirrors. I was not afraid. I was not aware of any sounds or pain or dizziness; it was like I was a fascinated viewer. When my spirit reached the height of about five feet, there appeared to be a "vapor like" substance swirling within my body. Like a twister the vapors formed a narrower, swirling column and rose upwards out of my back and past me out of my line of vision. A feeling of tremendous relief spread over me. The more the vapors flowed out, the better it felt. It was a fabulous feeling. When the volume of vapors exiting decreased, and I felt my spirit start to move down towards my back, I silently cried "no, no, that's not all of them." As my spirit re-entered my back I thought "there is still a little left." I had no idea how much time elapsed. When I again became aware of my surroundings, I was surprised to find I was soaking wet. I had sweated so much it was as if someone had thrown a bucket of water on me. My partner said something strange had just happened. What was it? I was too embarrassed to tell her, so I said, "I don't know."

I had never thought of an out-of-body experience, but if I had, I probably would have dismissed it as not possible. Neuroscientists have described the experience as "looking down at one's corporal self." Their theory is that this is a mild interruption in the multi-sensory regions of the brain communicating with each other. As part of their studies, they have simulated an experience in an epilepsy patient by applying mild electrical current to specific parts of her brain (N.Y. Times, October 2, 2006). There may be a scientific explanation, but I believe it was related to the emotional strain I had just experienced and was so out-of-character that I was too embarrassed to tell anyone. A short time later, when I visited my father, he asked a question that was completely out of character for him, of what I had been doing on the specific date and time of my out-of-body experience. Suspiciously, I asked "why?" He said, "At that time I was dancing and suddenly I felt our spirits meet in another plane." From an otherwise much grounded, factually-oriented person, this was shocking. Never before, and never again, would I ever hear anything even vaguely related to this type of experience from my father. But I knew what he meant and believed he was correct. A couple of days later, I snitched a book from his shelf to read on my airplane ride home. At 30,000 feet I read in Jonathan Living Seagull the story of seagulls who meet in a "different plane." I got chills when I looked out the windows at the white clouds: was it a coincidence that it was Good Friday?

All these visuals must have been near the surface because they flew by in a nana-second as I thought of a response to the nurse's question: "Have you ever had an out-of-body experience?" My normal pattern would have been to dodge the question with an answer I refer to as a "passing" one meaning not a "yes" or "no," such as "why do you ask" or "what do you mean?" However, deciding that the few seconds before heart surgery was not the time to be evasive, my hesitant voice from the gurney said, "Yes."

Many times in my life I had generated unusual reactions in people: but nothing as unexpected as this one. I was quiet: so was she. Her facial expression was hard to read: mine showed surprise. I lay perfectly still: she started pushing my gurney towards the swinging doors. Just before we hit the doors, she leaned and whispered, "Then you'll be all right, it is not your time yet." Had my preparation or it being a Sunday helped?

CHAPTER 8. SUNDAY, JANUARY 14TH: HEART SURGERY

My body was still: my mind was trying to process her words, "Then you'll be all right, it is not your time yet."

Immediately after the words left her lips, she handed my gurney over to a set of waiting hands and left my world. As my gurney rolled towards the center of the room, the sides of my brain sprung into action. My emotional side screamed "that's great news." My analytical side said, "Yes if we can believe her."

The emotional side responded, "Why not believe her," to which the analytical side asked, "Do we have anyway of evaluating the truthfulness of her assurances?"

"She didn't have to say that we would be all right," said my emotional side. "Maybe she says that to everybody. Do you think she would really tell a person heading into heart surgery that his time had come?" responded the analytical side.

"Very few people have out-of-body experiences so why did she ask you that question?" "You have never told anyone about ours, so why did you tell her?"

"She saw, or felt, something that caused her to risk her job by even asking the question."

"What?"

"I don't know but I felt being wheeled into heart surgery was not a time to be coy," the emotional side replied as it switched to reasoning.

The analytical side replied, switching to emotions, "I agree that there must be something about us because even on the first meeting people tell us personal things that many times they have not even told their friends."

"Come on, do you really think this experienced surgical nurse would do that? What would we be thinking if she had said, "That's too bad, as your time has come'?" The analytical side replied, "That she was wrong; but I don't think she was."

"Isn't it better to be wondering if she was right rather than if she was wrong?" "Is there anything we are not considering?"

"Is it simply chance that it is Sunday?"

My gurney completed its journey to the "other" table; the one under the light. My right side screamed, "This is your last chance. Do not get on that table." My left side calmly replied, "Stop it. We have done all that we can to be ready;: it is time to have faith." From my carotid surgery only two days ago, I knew the next steps. I started to lift my left leg over my right in order to roll onto the "other" table. A voice said, "No, we will do that. Just lie still and we will lift you." I did, and they did. For the second time in three days a mask was put over my face without any accompanying instructions. So, again, I began my own count: 100, 99... 91... no sounds, no smells, no tastes, no sense of touch, no thoughts, no sense of time: nothing.

Part of my being ready was my understanding the procedure. The estimated time for my surgery was six to eight hours. The anesthesiologist would achieve a balance of slowing my blood flow down enough so the surgeon could work on my heart while keeping it beating fast enough so my organs remained alive. The brain does not store blood but it will atrophy, a polite word for cease functioning, after 3-5 minutes without blood. The surgical team had to ensure sufficient blood flow to keep the brain alive, but not enough to cause too much bleeding or loss of blood which, during the surgery, could also cause complications. My carotid surgery was performed before the heart surgery to reduce the risk of changes in my blood pressure causing plaque to break loose, circulate through my system and cause a stroke. It speaks to the skill of the surgeons that they are able to depend on my right carotid artery working less than two days after surgery to re-open it.

The seriousness of my surgery was illustrated by the projected length of six to eight hours as, according to the National Heart and Lung

Institute, traditional open heart surgery takes three to five hours. It begins with a six to eight inch incision down the center of your chest wall. Your ribs are broken and separated. A breathing tube is passed through your mouth into your lungs and connected to a ventilator, which helps you breathe during the surgery. How a patient breaths during the surgery can occur in one of two ways: The "traditional" way, is to steady your heart with a mechanical device so your blood never leaves your body. The other way is a heart-lung bypass machine connected to your heart to move the blood outside your body. Medicine is then given to stop your heart from beating. The machine removes carbon dioxide, adds oxygen and pumps the blood back into your body. Tubes are inserted to remove fluid from your chest. After the heart is repaired, the tubes are removed and medicine is given to start your heart beating again. Sometimes a mild electrical shock is needed to restart your heart.

My surgeon had told me that he preferred the traditional way as outlined by the National Heart and Lung Institute. He had said that no matter how careful he was, and in surgery he was very careful, anytime the blood was removed from your body the risk of infections was increased. Before the surgery, he felt that my being in reasonably good physical condition gave him hope that he could avoid having to use the heart-lung machine.

My surgery was referred to as a "bypass," which is where the blockage in my arteries is "bypassed" so the blood can flow around the blockage; i.e., by-pass it. My surgery was typical in that the material for the bypass was constructed from my veins. My left leg was opened from just above my knee to my ankle and a vein removed to be used for my bypasses. Veins are amazing. They have "one way valves" which permits the flow of blood towards the heart while preventing it from flowing back the other way. Arteries do not have these valves, so the vein removed must be "stripped" of the valves. The veins are cut into pieces and attached on each side of the clogged portion of the arteries. In this way the blood can bypass the blockage and continue to supply the body with blood. In a bypass, the veins are placed on the outside of the arteries, while stents are placed inside the arteries to ensure the blood can continue to pass.

During surgery, time is crucial for the surgical team. The anesthesiologist had estimated putting me under the anesthetic for eight hours. But all eight hours would not be the same. The anesthetic must be administered to reduce the shocks to my body. It takes considerable skill to ensure that I "go under" and "come out" slowly. Coming out too quickly would put me in great danger, which I think of as being like the danger of the "bends" (Caisson's disease) that happens when an underwater diver rising too quickly to the surface from a deep dive destroys the balance of between the nitrogen in our bodies and the surrounding substances, be it water or air. When the pressure of one changes, like when a diver goes deep or a patient's blood slows, the body must be given time to make the adjustment. Insufficient time causes us to have a nitrogen solubility problem (an "aero-embolism") that will cause serious brain damage.

At the completion of my surgery, wire was used to bind my ribs together, along with staples and stitches to close my chest. In the recovery room the anesthesiologist was planning to prevent a nitrogen problem by controlling my rate of returning to consciousness. This was so routine that he permitted Carol to stand in the tiny room. However, as I had been, and would continue to be, I was an exception to any routine! This time the first sign was when I started moving my hands much sooner than expected, or planned, by the anesthesiologist. This anesthesiologist, skilled at controlling the process for patients of varying physiology, through hours of carefully making micro adjustments, knew my hands moving meant I was returning too quickly: hours too quickly. For some reason, which I believe was my will to live, I was coming out of the anesthetic so fast that it surprised and scared the experienced anesthesiologist. He had to do something---now--- to stop my hands from moving: if he failed there was a high risk of brain damage.

He ordered Carol out of the room. While she watched through the glass window, he tried methods to slow my recovery: they failed. Out of desperation, the anesthesiologist defied procedures by asking (ordering?) Carol to return to the recovery room. Carol pushed herself off the wall she had been leaning against to prevent her propensity to faint, and somehow, someway, managed to put my health in front of her own and re-entered the recovery room. She, with no medical training except what comes from being a mother of two active boys, looked at the anesthesiologist and his eyes said it all: she had to act. She said, "He hates to have anything in his mouth," as she watched my right hand try to reach towards my mouth to remove the breathing tube taped in my mouth. The anesthesiologist said it was vital that it remain in my mouth. Carol took over. She quietly, calmly explained to me, "The tube has to stay in your mouth and if you don't stop trying to pull it out, they are going to have to tie your hands down again." She knew about the only thing I hated more than a tube in my in mouth was having my hands tied.

Suddenly within my closed eyes a visual appeared. It was row after row of white framed shadow boxes on a black background, tilted slightly higher on the right side, slowly rolling from the bottom of my sight to the top. Each of the endless rows had five identical boxes. Each box contained a glowing, three dimensional, very lifelike version of Carol's head with her mouth saying something I could not hear. They were terrifically comforting. I was aware of immediately feeling peaceful. I relaxed, moved my right hand, yes I was aware that it was my right hand reaching for my mouth, to my side and stopped moving my hands while returning to nothingness.

Later, when I opened my eyes, I was incredibly happy! I was alive. I could see. I was woozy and had no thoughts except relief that I was alive. This was really all that mattered.

I later learned of the scenario with the anesthesiologist and that Carol's help had been crucial in returning me to consciousness at the right pace. I like to think it was the strength of my spirit that surprised the anesthesiologist by fighting for consciousness sooner than he expected. Did it help during the surgery? Did it almost cause brain damage by causing me to defy the skills of the anesthesiologist? Did the pre-op nurse know something? Could it being a Sunday have made the difference?

CHAPTER 9. MONDAY, TUESDAY:
JANUARY 15, 16:
HEALING MYSELF?

Monday: I am alive. I made it. I survived two major surgeries in three days. The surgeons, with help, cured me, were my first conscious thoughts Monday morning. My eye lids became very heavy as a wave of relief rolled through my stomach and spread down my legs. I was alive. I had a second chance at life. To me, these seven short words were the world's greatest message. I had not knowingly started the wave, nor could I stop it. I just enjoyed it. When it hit my toes, my mind let go and I drifted to somewhere peaceful.

My eye lids slowly opened but no other part of my body even thought of moving. It was a good thing because they could not have moved anyway. Heart surgery can do that to you; at least it did it to me. I smiled at Carol, or at least tried to smile. I saw the tubes and the stand holding the clear bags of liquid. There were so many of them it was unnerving. My eyes followed the tubes down and into a taped bandage on my right wrist. This did not scare me. I was alive. If this was what it took, then it was beautiful. I thought that it must be morning, although there were no windows in the Intensive Care Unit (ICU). Intensive Care, like casinos, was designed to keep the focus inward. There was nothing so important that it compelled me to challenge the soreness in my throat from the breathing tubes inserted through my mouth used during surgery.

A tall white haired man in a white coat entered and his ear-to-ear smile said it all even before he said those oh so sweet words, "Your bypass surgery went well." Dr. W continued, "I did five bypasses and did not have to use a cardiopulmonary bypass machine, sometimes called a heart-lung machine or simply a blood pump, so you will not need to use blood thinners. Let me have a look at your bandages." The effects of the anesthetics made it difficult to immediately process his words. Did he say five? His demeanor was easy. I loved his smile and enthusiasm. I looked down as he gently stooped and pulled my sheets back. My chest was completely bandaged. "It looks good," he said. "I stapled your ribs together." He pulled the sheet down farther and I saw that my left leg was bandaged from the knee down. "I took a vein from your leg to use for your bypasses." He checked the bags hanging from the stand and the bandages holding them onto my right wrist before he walked around my bed and did the same thing to the ones hanging on my left and attached to my left wrist. "Everything looks good," he said. "Just as I thought it would based on your overall health."

I was slowly processing his words. Everything looked good. My good overall health had helped. Thankfully, ever so thankfully, he did not have to use a blood machine. This was great news. Besides surviving, much of my pre-surgical mental focus had been on preventing the need for a blood machine. I took some pride knowing that I had done my part and maybe, just maybe, my efforts helped. Five by-passes sounded like a lot, but the full impact of the size of this number would not hit me until later when I would never meet anyone else who had so many. I knew I was alive. I was afraid to even think about a stroke, let alone ask about one. So I asked what I thought was an easy question, "Am I cured?"

Dr. W turned serious when saying, "I did what I could surgically. Now the rest is up to you. Your heart stopped because it was out of rhythm. We are now keeping it in rhythm but if your heart does not regain its rhythm on its own by tomorrow morning, I will have to do another procedure."

My face must have shown the shock before I could regain my breath and force my mouth to utter the words, "What? I thought you said the surgery was a success?"

"It was," he continued. "I did all that I said I would. I corrected the blockage around your heart which undoubtedly prevented a heart attack. You did not have a heart attack. During a heart attack part of your heart dies permanently, since a heart cannot re-grow itself. None of your heart died. Your heart got out of rhythm and shut down. Think of it like your heart having a timer, like for a watch or the metronome used to help the rhythm of piano players, that got so out of rhythm that it got over whelmed and just stopped. For the past five days we have assisted your heart in maintaining its rhythm while we dealt with your other problems. But this has to be temporary. Now we are going to remove the assistance. Your body must correct itself. In case it does not today, we are scheduling a procedure for tomorrow morning at 6 A.M. But our surgery was a success."

I felt his words permeating through my body, reversing the peacefulness I initially experienced. I had won the battles of two major surgeries in three days but still had not won the war. This reality left me emotionally drained and very weary: I needed to rest. But I couldn't. I needed to again focus. Now what did he say? I did not have a heart attack? If he had said that before, I did not process it, but I did now. In a heart attack part of your heart dies permanently. No part of my heart had died. I had not had one although the morning my heart stopped. My mind instantly replayed the events, as it would again and again: the morning, the drive to the clinic, the examination room and the technicians, striding towards the framed print on the wall while on the treadmill, the burning in my lungs as I gasped for breath while the technician sought on-the-job training on the machine, talking to the cardiologist, looking up at the blond lady with the moist cloth, the gurney ride, looking up at Carol, and all the other events surrounding my two surgeries. I remembered the numerous words of encouragement, and warnings, from the vascular surgeon, then the cardiac surgeon, "We will perform the surgery tomorrow morning, if you still qualify." I shuttered at the memories of my nights afraid that any movement might disqualify me and my chances for survival. Hours of darkness with my body screaming for the peace of sleep but my subconscious being afraid to let go because bad things happened to me when I was not on guard. Automatically, I had focused all my energies on winning the battles. For six rugged days, and nights, my mind had been fighting my body and the surgeons. Through two surgeries, and in-between, the surgeons had used anesthetics to slow my bodily processes down. They had done their job on my body, which now just craved rest. My body, and mind, were exhausted from all the news that had been steadily bombarding it that it could not fully comprehend. But comprehension would have to wait, as would the much needed rest. My mind had only one priority: to survive. This morning I thought I had fought as long as I could. Now I could, and must, rest. But instead I had to gear up to avoid another procedure, whatever it might be. Asking if I could find the strength never occurred to me: I simply would.

I wanted to learn the causes of heart problems. However, I automatically followed a lesson I had learned in my legal practice. I would start by asking clients to describe the effects in their own words. I would listen for legal issues without assigning labels, while drawing an imaginary time line to help differentiate the causes from the effects. "Effects" needed to be solved before the "causes." For the last six days in the hospital, I had devoted all my energies on fighting the effects. My relief was in thinking that I had won was interrupted by the news that I had another fight to prevent another procedure. I began to realize the similarities between the approaches of the legal and medical professions, who followed the same procedure of prioritizing the effects, my heart stopping, before alter addressing the cause(s).

I had found that the most difficult question to answer was the simple one word for peoples' actions: Why? In the beginning of my law practice, I would focus on why people did things. But as my practice grew, I had to continually search for ways to increase efficiencies. One way was to make clients feel more comfortable so they would share the information I needed to understand, and solve, their legal issues. Towards that end, clients needed to feel understood, which meant I had to provide them an opportunity to explain why they were in this situation. My challenge was to keep this explanation brief since while I always found the "why" interesting, it sometimes took so much time that it squeezed the time left to find a solution. This was illustrated when I practiced what I came to call "escalator" law, which was when a client would join me on the escalator in our building and expect to describe a situation and receive a legal opinion before we completed the two story ride. I learned during those rides to narrow the issues down to the necessary essentials, such as "what, where, when and how," all of which were admissible in court. Conspicuous by its absence was sometimes the most interesting question: why, since the answer was always subjective, meaning it was subject to challenge in court.

This provided a perspective for the type of questions to ask of a client in order to find a creative solution in a very limited time. My search led back to the law and the theory that someone is presumed to be responsible for their actions. So to initially solve the legal issues, I could just assume there was a "why." I was aware that since I had graduated law school there was a growing trend to expand the physical and psychological reasons why someone was not responsible for their actions. There are multiple views supporting, and opposing, this trend. The concern in my practice was always how potentially innocent victims could protect themselves from persons rather than ask if, and why, some were not legally responsible for their actions.

The top two philosophical answers to the theoretical question of "why" have been stated as "why not" and "because," both thoughtful but not very helpful for me in either my legal practice or in a hospital bed. So rest and the answer to why would have to wait. Now I had to focus on Dr. W. saying I had to correct myself. As they teach in journalism school, the essential parts of a story are answering the what, when and where questions, to which my legal training had taught me to add "how?" The " what" was survival, the "when" was now and the "where" was here. What was missing was where my creativity as an attorney started: How? I asked myself the same question that we frequently asked a witness: Have you taken anything that might alter your ability to think straight? My answer to this question was a definite "yes" as anesthetics make focusing difficult, and it takes time for them to completely leave our bodies. The time it takes varies with the quantities administered, and mine were huge, and the condition of the patient, and I was weak from my previous surgery just two days ago. The general rule is it takes at least 45 days for the anesthetics to leave our bodies, although some estimates are that it takes six months to completely leave. The drugs permeate not only our consciousness but cause our entire bodies to slow down. Our memories and energy levels are easy to identify, but what about our reasoning?

These thoughts confused and exhausted me. So, once again, I focused on effects by asking myself, "After what I have been through, is having a normal life worth one more day of fighting?" As in practicing law, the answer frequently was setting the context for the question, which in legal jargon was called "laying the foundation." The foundation for my question of "how" was that I was alive and lying in Intensive Care in a fine hospital, after having been seen, inspected, probed, measured, tested and monitored from head to toe. I had survived two major surgeries within three days, each preceded with the warning that I might not qualify. I had done my part to qualify and the surgeons had done their part of restoring the blood flow to my brain and heart. Our team efforts were rewarded. No part of my heart died. I did not have a stroke. I do not need blood thinners. I had defied the odds so great that when I thought of them, it was hard to believe it. I had come a long way. Now I needed to finish but the question of how needed to be answered.

I sought the help of a greater power. I hoped, argued (after all I am an attorney), prayed and focused all my consciousness toward my body healing itself. I was trying to unleash the power of my subconscious. I took deep breaths and visualized energies flowing from my neck down into my body. It sounds strange, but I felt them entering my chest and then flowing lower with my message "Body you are an amazing creation of our creator. You do so many things that I don't understand. When you sense a need to digest, process or cure, you respond. I need you to use your magic to cure my heart's rhythm."

The daytime flew by; the night did not. Every time my body overcame my mind and tilted my head, always to my left due to the bandages on my right carotid, I would jerk awake. The hands on the school house clock above my nurse had a mind of their own. Sometimes they raced and sometimes they crawled so slowly that the only way I could tell if they were moving at all was to watch the second hand. Tick, tock, went the clock; the large hand pushing the small one towards the top of its face and Tuesday and the start of the downhill run from 12 to 6 and the answer to "Was I cured?" It helps me to consider the worst possible result since knowing I can handle it usually helps me to relax. But this was not a usual time. I could not even imagine what would happen if I didn't cure myself and my fate depended on other procedure working.

Tuesday: The hands on the clock passed through midnight and Tuesday began. Not just any Tuesday, but the Tuesday of the dreaded procedure. The tubes and bandages provided part of the reason why I remained in a sitting position and my subconscious did the rest. I felt that

I needed to calm my heart in order to give it a chance to recover, so I tried a form of yoga. I visualized my heart muscles working perfectly and my mind cleared, my eye lids descended and my head slowly sank towards my left shoulder. Then my eyes jerked open and my head sprang back to the upright position with a speed that would make a chiropractor proud. My body needed rest but my mind was afraid to let go. The clock said 12:15 AM. Was there something I could be doing to correct my heart's rhythm? 12:30 AM: how many procedures could I take? 12: 45 AM: when would my luck run out?

I closed my eyes and tried to think of nothing. Even in yoga when instructors suggested that we think of a place that made us happy, while the other participants sighed in relief, my mind started arguing whether it was oceans or mountain streams. Now I realized it was neither: it was people. So I thought of family. Tick, tock; the clock striking one reminded me of the child's verse "the mouse ran up the clock, the clock struck one," and how clever we had felt at adding "and the rest got away."

At 2:05 A.M. my nurse, who never talked, said in a slow steady voice, "Your heart has corrected itself." These magical words filled my eyes with moisture. He continued, " You will not need the procedure if the correction holds." Uh oh, another "if I qualify." I tried to feel the difference in heart beats so I would be able to tell if I slipped back: no luck. I would not know until someone told me. So I continued to lie perfectly still. The only sound was my breathing. 4, 5, and finally 6 and no one came. Maybe they were just late. A nurse looking through the large window caused great apprehension before disappearing. My nurse was silent: so was I. What if they forgot and my asking reminded him of my procedure? At 7 A.M., Carol walked in and I whispered, "Have you heard whether my procedure is still scheduled?"

She looked surprised as she said, "Don't you know it was canceled?"

I said, "No, and I was afraid to ask. What was the procedure?"

"Didn't you know it was to be the paddles?"

A chill ran from my toes to my head: The paddles? Paddles carried electricity. Movies flashed before me: electricity makes the body jump, makes people think slowly when applied in therapy, paralyses people when used in a stun gun, and kills people strapped in electric chairs. The only time when the paddles were used on me, I was not breathing. What must they feel like when I would be conscious?

Unbeknownst to me at the time, our bodies always have electricity running through them as our nervous system uses it to communicate. The speed of electricity enables us to instantaneously respond to a stimulus, like a clear and present danger. The message from the brain is transferred by an electrical charge which runs from cell to cell. Any other means, like manual or chemical, would be far too slow for us to avoid dangers or otherwise promptly respond to a stimulus. The electrical impulses that regulate the heart originate from the mass of cells located in the right atrium that are called the "sinoatrial node," or simply the "SA node." Coronary artery disease, like mine, occurs when the arteries are so blocked that they cause a deprivation of oxygen which causes the SA nodes to constantly tell the heart to contract which, in turn, prevents it from ever fully contracting. The physicians were hoping, and I was praying, that once the blockages in my arteries were bypassed, the oxygen deprivation would be cured and my SA nodes would no longer be constantly sending messages to contract. In short, everything would return to normal. This was what happened at 2 A.M. on January 16th. If it had not, it was hoped that the paddles would "jump start" my SA nodes; analogous to jump starting a car.

I sat quietly enjoying the euphoria of the stress running down my body and out my toes. Was it all right to rest now? Had my body finished my healing? So many confusing thoughts, so much to share, all mixed together. Confusion overwhelmed me and my mind gave in to fatigue.

When I woke, my mind was now free to begin to notice my surroundings. My hospital room was relatively spacious and painted in an off-white color with yellow or green tinting, depending on the glare from the florescent lights. By looking straight ahead I could see through my only window into the hallway, which was where I had traded glances with the nurse who I thought might be coming for me. The wall on my left was just far enough away for someone to have access to my left side. On my right there was a padded chair and a desk near the door where my personal nurse sat under a small desk light writing. Discovering my surroundings felt good after days of lying quietly while things were done to, and for, me by people wearing white or green coats. I appreciated the ones who politely used the first person plural pronoun "we" rather than the pronoun "you." Oh, I knew I was alone in the bed I had "discovered" the difference in attitude of my clients, and maybe even me, when I switched from saying what "you" are going to do to what "we" are going to do when discussing legal alternatives. Using the pronoun "we" indicated that we were a team. Of course my clients understood there were limits to this theory but, fortunately, I did not practice criminal law where the differences might come at the jail house door.

My bandages limited my ability to see a nurse when she walked past my head and out of my line of vision. The unknown was always a mystery. Where was she going? What was behind the headboard of my bed? I remembered the curiosity created when my eyes were taped shut for a week after eye surgery. I must have dozed as my eyes opened to a nurse saying, "It is time to stand up." My body wanted to just lie still. My mind always tries to remember that the medical folks were my team mates who wanted to prevent the many post surgical problems caused by the lack of movement. Even with the knowledge that muscle atrophy can start after just three days, I didn't think my body was capable of moving. The nurse adjusted my intravenous tubes; first the three on my right then the three on my left, keeping them from tangling. She encouraged, actually required, me to roll my left leg over my right one. The nurse helped, as in picking up and moving my legs over the side of the bed, which pulled my trunk into a sitting position. After a short rest, the nurse guided me up into my first standing position in a week. I was not dizzy (for a medical description of this procedure see uchospitals.edu). She encouraged my two steps to the padded cloth chair where I was expected to sit: but how? Sitting down would require the use of my stomach muscles, which I could not do, so I just flopped down. As any woman will verify, flopping down in a very short skirt can require some rearranging. I was unable to even rearrange my hospital gowns which must have been designed by someone with either a sense of humor or revenge for those of us bigger than petite. Modesty even creeps in when it was only the nurse and me in an Intensive Care Unit.

The nurse said, "Time to walk." Her tone reminded me of my mother saying "Rise and shine," during my junior high days. Then I would mumble, "I will rise, but I will not shine." Today I just groaned. I knew walking, or more properly shuffling, was important to prevent post surgery circulatory problems, as well as muscle atrophy. A lack of motion can cause the blood flow to be sluggish or slow causing blood clots deep in veins for a condition known as Thrombosis (nim.nih.gov). Athletes know the importance of continuous exercise, hence the origin of the phrase "use it or lose it." I had always taken my ability to walk for granted. What I was about to learn was that I would have to relearn many of the bodily functions. I began to appreciate what infants, and their bodies, go through. Infants smile, giggle and bounce on their first steps: I did not. Unlike infants, my thoughts got in the way. I was weak and unsteady and afraid that if I fell, the needles sticking in me would twist and break. I remember being in a line in the induction center for the army when an orderly, to draw blood, walked down the line and stuck a needle in each person's left arm while saying, "Hold this with your right hand." Apparently I wasn't the only one to be surprised at how warm the blood was: I heard thumps from the men fainting with the needles still in their arms. On this first walk in seven days I pushed my I.V. stand all of 40 feet, which was as far as I could and still get back. My walk reminded me that I had also had major surgery on my left leg. All the nurses turned their heads and smiled as I passed, which I took as encouragement. Later I wondered if it had anything to do with the open back to my under sized gown. My reflection in the window to the nurses' station showed me to be so feeble that I was glad that Carol was not there to see her "protector" barely able to walk.

Carol had moved to a more private, quiet area of the hospital for a work related conference call. Her pale look when she returned caused a nurse to ask, "Are you all right?" Carol said "yes," but her posture said "no." Carol was the only employee who could do her job, which had to be done. So her boss phrased it this way, "You can take time to visit your husband, as long as you keep up with your work load." Of course her work load normally required ten hour days of constant motion.

My day was one of emotionally and physically resting thinking my surgeries and procedures were over: or were they?

CHAPTER 10. WEDNESDAY, THURSDAY: JANUARY 17, 18: MANAGING HOSPITAL PROCEDURES

Wednesday: On my eighth hospital day, my first thought was, "Will this be my first day in an Intensive Care Unit without a scheduled surgery or procedure?" An Intensive Care Unit (ICU), also known as Intensive Therapy Unit or Intensive Treatment Unit or Critical Care Unit (CCU) is a special part of a hospital that provides intensive medicine (Wikipedia). Admission is based on a physician finding that close observation or specialized monitoring and/or therapy is necessary (health communities.com). It is designed to not stimulate our senses. There are no sunrises, no sunsets, just florescent lights whose flickering we learned in graduate school was harmful to our eyes. It is never too hot, too cold, or too much anything. The occasional sounds of service were the only interruptions to the ever present hum of florescent lights. Even the smell of the food never changed much meal-to-meal. In the past week nothing changed: except me, albeit very slowly. Now there were times when my eye lids were no longer too heavy to lift when I felt the presence of someone, even those who checked my bandages, lifting my wrist to look at the contraption that holds the tubes, flicking their fingers on the tubes, clearing bags hanging on the pole, or bringing me things I had not ordered or wanted, like needles. When a white coat took my temperature by rubbing a hand held measuring device over my forehead, my body was passive but my mind smiled at the progressions the taking of temperatures had taken from the days when it had begun with the dropping of my shorts, through glass thermometers filled with mercury stuck in my mouth that if I bit down would be fatal, to things being stuck into my ears, to today. Today, Wednesday, my mind had the luxury of having these thoughts.

While feeding myself breakfast, which I now could, I inadvertently winched when Dr. W., my cardiac surgeon, entered. As he checked my bandages, he said with a smile, "Everything looks fine." Great words but I knew the routine. I silently waited for the punch line, the line where he would describe my new qualifying challenge. This day, this beautiful Wednesday, he had none.

I drifted peacefully into, and out of, consciousness. It was wonderful. It is important to get enough rest after heart surgery (ClevelandClinic.org) so our bodies can use its energies to heal. Sometime in the morning a nurse told me it was time to sit in my chair. Having done this before, I had plenty of time to think about my part as she carefully organized the tubes running from the rack to my arm, pulled my blanket back, my gown down, and made me feel proud when I did my two parts: sliding my left leg over my right one and standing, of course with her help. I noticed how effective she was at handling me. Critical Care nurses have received specialized training and provide round the clock bedside monitoring and care (healthcommunities.com).

Once in the chair, I saw the mystery of where the nurses went when they walked behind my bed: nowhere. My bed was against the wall. What a reminder of how small my world had become. I love dogs and I smiled, I think, when a large dog walked over and put his nose in my lap. I tried to raise my hand to pet him: I could not. Disappointingly I said, "Thanks for bringing him and please bring him again but now I am too weak to pet him." I have loved dogs since the day before starting kindergarten when my father brought home a Dalmatian. My choice of "Spot" as a name lost to Gallant. In recent years I had learned the value of therapeutic dogs in lowering anxiety, stress, and heart and lung pressure among heart failure patients (American Heart Association).

The nurse smiled while saying, "It is time for our walk." My family has always said that my face showed my feelings, but if they showed through all the bandages, the nurse ignored them. A voice rang in my head saying, "If you want to recover, you have to walk." But if I started to fall, could I trust her to catch me? Of course not, but to recover I sort of had to trust. It was only "sort of" because part of my recovering was to regain responsibility for myself. As I walked I was looking for things I might grab if I started to fall. This was a slow start, but it was a start.

Wednesday's highlights---eat, medicine dose, walk, eat, dose, talk to Carol---would only count as highlights in an ICU but it was my first day in the ICU without worrying about a surgery or procedure.

Thursday: On Thursday, after breakfast a nurse announced, "It is moving day." I was surprised even though I probably should have been thrilled as "Once close observation or specialized therapies are no longer required, the patient is discharged from ICU to a regular room or a concentrated care unit where modified care or therapy can be administered" (healthcommuniites.com). With the usual help, I got into a wheel chair and rolled down the hall and around the corner, the mystery corner since it was beyond my walks. Now there was no mystery to what lay around it: more hospital hallways. As my wheel chair entered my first non-intensive care room in over a week, I smiled at seeing the sun. As soon as the attendant pulled the cover backs, moved me from chair to bed, lifted my legs, arranged the pillows, adjusted the bed and pulled the covers up, I fell asleep.

When I opened my eyes, I saw circles of color that looked like balloons. They were balloons. Then I heard laughter. It was my friend Stan sitting next to my bed. His laugh was contagious. I had not known that I could still laugh, but it sure felt good. He handed me a package of Junior Mints, which I immediately recognized as a reference to the Seinfeld episode where Cramer and George wrestling while watching a surgery, caused a Junior Mint to go flying into the air where it landed inside the patient's surgically opened body. As could only happen in a Seinfeld episode, the surgeons, unaware of its presence, closed the patient with it inside him and, of course, this was only the beginning of problems. Stan's visit was cut short by my dosing but remembering the Junior Mint episode was another sign that I did not have stroke.

I woke to find a white-coat entering carrying a small, innocuous looking package while saying, "I have brought your Voldyne." He explained that if I ever wanted to take full breaths, I needed to manually re-expand my lungs one breath at a time by blowing into the rubber hose hard enough to cause the small red rubber ball to hit the top of the six-inch plastic tube in which it was encased. I compared the concept to the one used in the carnival game called, alternatively, "Test Your Strength," "High Striker," Strength Tester," or "Strongman Game." In those games the contestant, it was almost always a male, invariably kept paying to keep trying to prove his manhood by swinging the wooden mallet hard enough to force a ball upwards to ring a bell at the top. I remembered the rumor that the secret to ringing the bell was not in the strength but in the technique. But if there was a similar technique for ringing the figurative bell at the top of the Voldyne, I never found it.

The technique taught me was to take a deep breath and blow as hard and long as I could until the ball in the plastic tube rang the symbolic bell at the top. I visualized that all I had to do was hit the bell the first time and, like blowing up a balloon, and each subsequent time would become easier. I took a cautious breath and blew what I thought was just hard enough to ring the bell but not so hard as to rip the staples holding my chest together. The ball did not move.

"To take a deep breath, you must breathe through your diaphragm," the white-coat said. I watched his stomach protrude and wondered if I had ever breathed properly. He explained that the way to expand my lungs was to take a deep breath for the count of four, then holding it in your stomach, although at first it might be my chest, forcing your diaphragm to expand to provide room for your lungs to expand. Diaphragms are a domed shape muscle at the bottom of our rib cages. When breathing out our diaphragm relaxes and we can increase the speed of air exhaled by contracting our transverse abdominal muscles. Diaphragms also help stabilize our trunk and deep breathing increases its strength.

The better understanding of my body I was gaining by being inquisitive was extended to my surroundings when I noticed a before lunch routine of a white-coated male walking into my room, and without a word of explanation, withdrawing a small amount of blood from my finger, leaving, then returning a short time later to give me an injection. In a little over a half-hour I would start to feel queasy. Then after lunch was served, I would start to feel better. This time I asked, "What are you testing for, and what is the injection?" My questions had a dual purpose: I wanted to understand what was being done to me, and I wanted the white-coat to double check that the treatment was being matched with the right patient. I was starting to think like a lawyer.

"The test is for your blood sugar levels, and the injection is insulin," to which I replied, "I have never been a diabetic," based on my understanding that insulin was used to control diabetes. One use of injections of insulin is supplementing the insulin that is produced by our pancreas in regulating the carbohydrates and fat metabolism by causing skeletal muscles and fat tissues to absorb glucose from the blood (Wikipedia).

"Your doctor believes your food will be more beneficial if preceded by an injection of insulin. There should be no reaction if your meals are served with 30 minutes, which they always are."

"Within a half hour, I start to feel queasy. I can see my lunch in the hallway but you folks are so busy that it is not served until much later. I thought about getting it myself but I am too weak. I am not agreeing to the injection."

"If you don't agree to the injection, I will tell your doctor."

"Tell him: he works for me," I said somewhat exaggerating while buying time to process the reasoning. "Let's try this: you take your test and then return with the injection after my tray has been served. I will wait for you before I take a bite." He did, I did, and I received the insulin without any queasiness. However, on this day I still was not hungry and I was unaware that lack of hunger, just like excessive hunger, maybe a warning sign of problems somewhere in the digestive system. But, like sleep, I was told that I needed to eat to recover.

I was still so weak that when my sheet or pillow became wrinkled, I had to lie on the wrinkles and wait for help. I could roll slightly to my left, or right, but not sit up. My new room had a television with a remote attached to a short cord running up from the floor. So short that it only reached the edge of my bed. If one of my few movements knocked it off, I had to leave the station and volume unchanged until someone retrieved it. Carol, perhaps motivated by my frequent requests, solved this small, but annoying, problem by tying the cord to the raised safety rails on the side of my bed.

A nurse arrived and announced, "You should have had a bowel movement by now." My similarities with childhood were continuing as someone else was keeping track of my not having one in a week. She continued, "We have been trying to stimulate one with diet but it hasn't worked. Try to have one but you should not strain as you might break your chest open; tomorrow we will try pills and if necessary, on Saturday, they would do a medical procedure." This was a grim reminder of how desperate I was. My mind raced into the conclusion that the dose of anesthetic that had to be so great that the surgeon could treat my heart, also impacted other parts of my body so much that these parts had to relearn how to function. My having to relearn breathing and walking seemed to fit this theory, so I guessed my lack of appetite was due to my system not having yet relearned how to digest and process food. Ultimately, I was scared of another procedure.

In the early evening, Carol arrived from work looking exhausted. My hospital week had taken its toll on her. She needed sleep and while feeling guilty I still needed her company. I felt very threatened by my latest problem and potential procedure. We compromise by her agreeing to stay with me until I fell asleep. She dosed and woke at 2 A.M. to leave. She was expected at work by 8. At the parking garage, she said to the attendant, "I have been visiting my husband, but I forgot to get my parking ticket validated. Will you please let me out? Between my job and the hospital, I have not had a chance to stop at the bank. Can I use a credit card?"

She tried a variety of alternatives including paying some maximum amount on a credit card, but the attendant insisted that she return to the hospital to have the ticket validated. This tactic threw her over the delicate edge she had been walking. She re-parked her car, returned to the hospital and started walking the halls looking for someone, anyone, who might be able to validate her parking ticket at 2 A.M. She finally found one woman who could validate the ticket.

The next morning, when it was obvious that she was upset (stress tends to magnify the impact of otherwise small problems), her boss asked why. After she described the garage incident, he reached into his pocket and loaned her a garage pass provided to him as a member of the hospital board as even hospitals have a hierarchy.

CHAPTER 11. FRIDAY, SATURDAY: JANUARY 19 & 20: ANOTHER MEDICAL PROCEDURE TO DIGEST?

Friday: My saying "Why so early?" caused the nurse's head and shoulders to jerk up and her half completed step to remain that way. It was evident that she was not used to patients being awake when she entered their rooms at 4 A.M., for her routine blood sample. But I had been awake for hours as per my hospital routine. Following my recently resumed "lawyer like" approach, I repeated, "Why so early?" Her facial expression showed the annoyance confirmed by her tone while saying, "Your doctor is very demanding. He insists all patients' tests be current and their files be complete and on his desk when he arrives at 6 A.M." In deference to her being armed with a needle, I moderated my thoughts by only saying, "being prepared sounds good to me."

Later my cardiac surgeon, Dr. W., who always arrived without any files but fully current, said, "I understand you had a discussion with a staff member." I was surprised that he knew, but his smile indicated that he was not upset. In ICU not upsetting your cardiac surgeon seemed like a good rule. "I told her I was thrilled that you were a perfectionist," to which he replied "I am afraid I am a dying breed." This so surprised me that I blurted out, "Why?" Pausing while taking a step backwards at this unusual twist in a conversation with a patient, he asked, "What do you do for a living?"

When I said, "I am an attorney who primarily represented

businesses in employment matters," he smiled while saying, "You must be busy." His posture stiffened and his smile disappeared as he related that recently he had written, in an abbreviated form, an unusual size dose for a drug on the top of an order form. Since this was one tenth the standard dose, to reduce the risk of an error by a nurse, he also wrote an unabbreviated version in the center of the form. A nurse filed a complaint alleging his repeating the dose was demeaning. The hospital human resources department had required that he take time from treating patients to write a response and then attend a meeting where the human resources employee told him to apologize. My internal red flags started frantically waving. I said that if I had represented him, I would have asked, "Why is double checking not a standard policy? Where was the greater duty of a doctor, nurse and hospital: to a patient or to an employee? Putting on my lawyer hat, the person primarily responsible, and liable, for treating a patient is their physician. If the wrong dosage was administered, the first question a lawyer would ask would be 'did the physician do everything possible to assist a busy nurse in not making an error'?" I felt sorry for the doc but it felt good to talk about something besides my health.

On his way out the door the surgeon paused, turned and said, "You seem like a thoughtful guy. Thoughtful people have much more trouble with the mental side of recovery." The meaning of his comment would puzzle, and haunt, me for a long time.

The nurse who brought the pills to stimulate my bowels arrived with a warning: if these do not work today, tomorrow we will use a procedure. The pills were welcomed as my stomach felt bloated and was hurting. I really was experiencing a new childhood. Within a week I had learned how to have my heart keep beating in proper timing, breathe, walk, chew, swallow and digest food, and now I had to learn how to complete the digestive process. Once again, I would have loved to know how to make my body comply. I continued to be amazed at how many things my body just automatically did without my knowing how. As the day progressed, so did the pains. The nurse also said, "You cannot leave the hospital until progress is made." I forced myself to do all that I knew might help: I drank some water.

A man and woman entered my room and the man said, "I'm with Mended Hearts. We are an organization of folks who have survived heart problems. We visit heart patients to offer encouragement from one who has also been there. I had a heart attack." He then described, in detail, his family, his job at a retail store near the pier, the day of his heart attack, the attack and life after his attack. His greatest message was his enthusiasm. I said, "Thank you for coming and sharing." I appreciated his efforts even though listening exhausted me and I was distracted by the potential procedure tomorrow morning. I decided to delay any decision about the organization, which I later would join.

A woman wearing a white coat walked in and said, 'Hi, I am the nurse from the cardiac rehabilitation center in the clinic. I am here to tell you about our rehabilitation program. We will monitor you continuously while encouraging you to gradually increase your physical activities." Her demeanor was understated with one exception, and it was a big one: her eyes. When she spoke, her words conveyed the script and her eyes enthusiasm. I thought of the program as an opportunity to push my limits in a controlled setting: in my lingo it was "fail safe."

I had mixed feelings about support groups. I appreciated the importance of sharing feelings and ideas with others. When my wife Anne was ill, I was approached to join a support group for spouses of those fighting cancer. The format was that the participants would take comfort from sharing their feelings. However, none of the other participants' worked ten hour days while trying to be a supportive spouse, father and home owner. I knew sharing was important and listening to the other members describe their problems might help them: but it would be deadly for me. My nature and training was to empathize with them but at the same time feel frustrated at not being able to solve their problems while keeping the responsibility for my own. Any "extra" time I needed to use to briefly escape my stresses.

On the other hand, a group that would help me focus on returning to life rather than discussing why, or where, I was, would be helpful. I developed a criterion: consider joining organizations that focus on the future and avoid those that focus on the past. I also categorize programs as short or long term. For short term you do whatever it takes to survive. Long term you do not completely recover from something until you spend most days not thinking, either positively or negatively, about it. For example, I felt I would never be "cured" of part of my addiction to sweets until I could pass a Dunkin Donuts Shop without even thinking about stopping.

My Friday in the hospital passed, but my waste did not. Midnight arrived with a reminder that my time was short to avoid another procedure. The pain from being bloated, and the fear of another unknown procedure, drove me to waddle over to the small bathroom in my room. I squeezed myself into the tiny space by putting my left arm on the sink and my right arm half way up the wall and waited, and waited, and waited. I was determined. In my groggy haze I realized how little I knew about the process. At 1:30 A.M. I decided to risk the stitches and strain: first gently and then hard. Maybe, maybe, I felt something very big moving slowly, very slowly, somewhere in my system. It seemed to take forever. How many feet of intestines do we have? This felt like a long trip as the pain moved first right-to-left before reversing itself. . Finally, it felt as if I had passed something bigger than the state of Delaware, where I used to live: maybe something as big as Maryland. Sorry, Delaware and Maryland, I hope you will forgive my moment of delirious, humorous relief.

After sitting for hours I could not get up. The white-coated woman arrived annoyed that I had rung the emergency button, and said, "It is not my duty to help you," I replied, "If you are embarrassed, imagine me, a 60-something year old attorney who can't get off the commode. Get over it and help me." To her credit she did. Had she not prevented me from following my childhood training, I would have flushed the marble sized evidence the specialist said he would need if there was any hope of avoiding the procedure. I fell asleep wondering if my renewed experience with Delaware would be sufficient to head off tomorrow's potential procedure.

Saturday: Saturday morning arrived as did the specialist in digestive issues. He walked in smiling and immediately answered my question of what would make this type of specialist smile, with, "Well, congratulations. I understand last night you had a movement. So we will not need a procedure." This news made me smile. Later I would learn that I was right to dread a procedure as, at least one of them, involved a manual insertion.

What a week of discovery. My body learned how to use my right carotid artery to distribute blood to my brain. My heart learned how to use the renewed flow of blood through my by-passes as well as how to regulate its own rhythm. I was learning how to properly breathe. My body "re-discovered" how to cut, chew, swallow without pain, digest and distribute the nourishment while disposing of the rest; while also learning how to distribute the blood in my left leg after the vein was removed. Two things stood out. One, I did not have to direct my body as it magically just somehow did it without my knowing how, and two, a new appreciation of what must be going on inside babies while they appear so helpless. I was healing under the bandages on my throat, chest and leg. Not visible was the healing of my carotid and ribs. My heart is a story unto itself. The surgeons removed a vein from my leg, stripped it of its one way valves, and attached it to my heart in five places. Taking one of my veins eliminated the chance of my body rejecting them. My heart then found its own rhythm. Sleep permitted my body to direct its energies to repairing me rather than burning it for movements. I was learning about life.

My cardiac surgeon entered, introduced his companion as the cardiologist on duty, before smiling and saying, "You have a choice. You can go home today or tomorrow."

I asked the cardiologist on duty and Carol what they thought. The cardiologist said, "Oh no, you are not putting me in that position." I was stunned. I could accept a "yes, no or maybe," but not the professionals equivalent of "It's not my job, man." My thoughts were "Then why are you here?" Carol's words "It's your decision" were reassuring but in contrast to the weariness in her eyes and shoulders.

My words of "I will stay another day" surprised even me since no one voluntarily stays in a hospital, but the immediate relief in Carol's eyes verified my intuition that Carol needed a day of rest and preparation. Tomorrow I will go home. Usually once I make a mental decision, such as leaving, I start preparing for the physical follow through. I learned the concept of mentally doing something before physically doing it from attorney Joe C., who had "mentally" resigned at 30,000 feet on his way to another country to respond to allegations of fraud by someone else that might land him in prison in a third world country. Shortly after returning, he physically resigned.

However, rather than plan ahead on this Saturday, I reflected on last Saturday when I had reviewed my life to avoid thinking about the surgery, and to start on a plan to learn what to change in rebuilding my life. I smiled at some memories and shuttered at others, but learned from both of them. How fast the sixty odd years had passed! I saw the error in my always driving for perfection. It had tended to focus me more on the on the smaller picture, the details of what could have been done better, rather than the larger, more important, aspects of life. I needed to change the very way that I thought of things and stop being an "internal stress generator." To do this I needed to become less a perfectionist. I remembered a saying I heard years ago: focus on the right things we do, rather than the wrong things, because the list is much shorter. Now this quip seemed to have meaning. Spending my potentially last day that way would turn out to be tremendously beneficial.

I began to feel a sense of accomplishment. I had achieved my short term goal of surviving and I was leaving the hospital with no permanent restrictions. When I think about leaving a hospital, I remember the lesson I learned at age seven: your condition when you leave a hospital is at least as important as when you leave. After having both my eyes bandaged shut for a week after eye surgery, I was jealous that Jimmy, who I never saw, was going home a day before me. Then I learned that besides being there five times, and scheduled to return, he might never recover from the steel splinter. Jimmy, yes I still remember his name, I have been rooting for you for over 60 years.

My breathing remaining a challenge was reminding me of what I, and others, would have given for a deep, clean breath of fresh air, when fighting asthma or bronchitis, as my children had, or pneumonia,a s I had. Why would anyone smoke of otherwise restrict their breathing?

It was obvious that the physical side of recovery was, and would continue to be, tough, but less obvious was the mental-emotional side, as predicted by the cardiac surgeon, would be just as tough. My wrestling with finding a way to manage the physical and mental-emotional aspects of rehabilitating-to-recovery is what led to "Managing Your Rehabilitation Program WELL."

A year later my sister Jill said, "I am surprised that you never once asked: why me." What a great illustration of addressing the issues in a sequence, beginning with stopping the effects. There would be time later to address the "why" question.

CHAPTER 12. SUNDAY, JANUARY 21:
GOING HOME AGAIN

<u>Sunday</u>: On Sunday, January 21, 2007, as had become my habit in the hospital, I woke wondering what would be my problem-of-the-day, and there always was one. After dodging yesterday's problem, that of a manual insertion in an unmentionable part of my body, I started trying to relate to the still somewhat threatening reality of going home again. For the past eleven days I could depend on a team of competent professionals to everything for, or to, me. The thought of my dependency ending was causing me to experience a mild version of the psychological phenomenon where a person becomes so dependent on one, or more, people that they become comfortable with the relationship and don't want it to end. For example, even in the extreme cases of being forcefully held as hostages, the FBI statistics show that 8% of hostages have experienced empathy and sympathy toward their captors. This phenomenon, called the "Stockholm Syndrome," was named after the bonding of captives with their capturers during a bank robbery in Stockholm Sweden. If 8% of hostages have these feelings after being traumatized, what percentage of hospital patients must have similar ones after being treated well?

I was going home for the first time in my second life! The reality of my helplessness was driven home when I tried to bend over to put on my first underwear in 12 days: socks were out of the question. We, my wheel chair pusher and me, rolled down the hallway so fast it added perspective to how short my "long" walks had been. This time the laughing that had followed my open backed gown walks was replaced by the good luck waves. As the lobby's sliding glass doors silently closed behind my wheel chair, I was reminded of the feeling of freedom that came when the heavy steel door closed behind me when I was leaving my law school legal clinic duties at the Brushy Mountain maximum security prison. For months afterwards, mostly late at night, I could hear that heavy metal prison door slamming behind us as we left. Those visits haunted me with thoughts of how those men, most of whom were my age, would be spending that, and many more, nights: what could possibly be worth that? I entered the prison wondering how I could defend myself while alone in an office giving counsel to the prisoners. I needn't have worried. They were all so normal: attentive, polite, soft spoken and reasonably articulate. One asked me to review a draft of a petition to a court that was so well done that I asked who had drafted it. He said, "I paid another prisoner a carton of cigarettes." This "jail house lawyer" would have been able to charge a lot more on the outside. I can still hear the voice of one prisoner objecting to being sent to solitary confinement for allegedly stealing his roommate's shirt, saying "Where does he think I was going with it---I am serving a life sentence for murder." What vivid lessons in the importance of being responsible for your actions.

Leaving the hospital and getting into my vintage, a nice word for old, Jaguar, which was so low it must have been made in the days when men were shorter, gave me an indication of my future. Even the most basic movement required planning before slow motion execution. Were the wheels on my chair locked? Do I put weight first on my left or right leg? Which leg goes into the car first? I did not want to use my left one at all because of the surgery to remove the vein. Wait, the car was close to the curb. Why did the valet park it so close? Do I put my right foot in the street or on the curb? Can I bend my head down far enough to miss hitting it on the low door? Now twist, duck, swing into the car, and twist into the seat. I quickly realized that there would be no simple activities. It reminded me of the course I taught in "time and motion" study, where every motion was broken into so many composite parts that listing each one even for something as basic as standing up filled an entire page.

Seeing my wheel chair driver waiting for the next patient

stimulated a silent "thanks" to the vascular surgeon, cardiac surgeon, technicians, nurses, therapists, orderlies, food preparers and deliverers, and all those volunteers who had so liked my gown. There were a like number behind the scenes keeping the facilities in working order.

At home the more immediate tasks fell on Carol, such as the hospital's instructions labeled Open Heart Surgery-Home Care Instructions sheet. There were 52 different directions divided into groups with 3 directions for medications, 11 for incision care, 8 for when to call my doctor, 7 for diet tips, 20 for activities and 3 for stocking care. For me this might as well have been instructions for the Rubik Cube. I had no hope of complying without help. As detailed as it was, this list was nowhere near complete. I was on my own for learning how to walk, talk, stand, sit, sleep and shower. Every movement was so difficult that it was preceded by a few questions: Is it necessary? Will I be able to it? Will straining help or hurt my recovery? What will happen if I start but can't finish? I knew my physical movements were greatly impacted and would only later learn that so were my mental ones.

My having taught industrial engineering made me all too aware that life's functions had to be redesigned. In the morning, Carol would help me get into my "position-for-the-day," which was sitting on the end of the couch by the sliding glass doors. Removing the vein made raising my left leg very difficult but necessary as Carol, perched on a stool, strained to push an elastic stocking over my swollen left leg. With talcum powder the task remained difficult, but doable. This would exhaust me and my part was only to hold my leg up. Carol would put my "tools" close to me: the remote for the television, something to read and a glass of water. I even made space for my adversary, the Voldyne, since I knew I had to frustrate myself three times a day. On my first trip to the bathroom, I felt weak but the call of nature can be a strong motivator.

At bed time, one slow six-inch step at a time I moved to the near side of the bed. I partly slid, partly rolled, and partly flopped, into a sitting position knowing that any wrinkled sheet would remain that way. I tried to slide down but my breathing became much more difficult in any position other than straight up. To keep from rolling on me, Carol laid down on the couch. This lasted about a half hour before I called, "I am lonely." After being alone in the hospital bed, I was willing to trade some physical risks for emotional comfort. I continued to relax—sort of—but each time I dozed off my head dropped to the left causing it to jerk back upright. Even at home, sleep continued to be a problem no matter how tired I felt. Nothing worked, not even my tried and true method of turning on the television. I quickly found that in my second life my tastes had changed. World news was too remote; local news too personal. I no longer enjoyed any show where someone got hurt, even though I knew it was fiction. Love stories were more appealing, except when someone made a big deal out of something trivial, or made statements like "I would rather be dead." I would say to the screen, "you don't realize what you are saying." Sports were good as long as there were no injuries, even to an opponent. Medical shows, particularly the show about the recalcitrant genius, Doctor House, became too personal when, precisely 26 minutes into each episode, someone would get the paddles. The ideal program not only fit these criteria but also was interesting enough to hold my attention, but not so interesting that I wanted to stay awake. My heightened emotional state clearly influenced my opinions.

I have always liked breakfast. Now the caffeine in coffee stimulated my thoughts and helped, but not completely solved, my lack of adrenaline. Heart surgery greatly reduces our body's ability to produce adrenaline, which plays a key role in our ability to generate energy to either "fight or flight." I felt the stimulus but was unable to respond.

If there was any doubt about how dependent I was, getting my first shower in thirteen days eliminated it. Carol did everything except get wet: she adjusted the water in our stand up shower and helped me take off my pajamas. To step over the four inch step into our shower, I held onto the shower door: mistake. When the door slid, so did I. Bam, it hit the wall right before I hit it. But I did not fall. The floor was slippery, so I grabbed what I could, which was the soap holder. I gained an appreciation for the importance of the safety devices, such as handles. The shower felt so good! I was enjoying it so much that I felt sorry for those people who did not have this "luxury." Stepping out of the shower, I grabbed the towel rack for support. Wrong, again. It ripped off the wall. Previously, I would have been upset if anyone, including me, had ripped it off the wall. Having problems was teaching me a great deal about perspective. I would quickly learn another lesson as I stood there shivering. Heart patients can have trouble with temperature differences. The room temperature was fine. It was me. I could not tolerate any chill.

It took more than 15 minutes under a thick blanket to stop shaking.

After the elastic stockings, my clothing choices came down to things that would go on easily. My new uniform of the day was shorts with an elastic top and a tee shirt. The preparations for each of my three walks a day took longer than the walks. I would stand like a boxer preparing to enter the ring as Carol placed my new, silky robe over my shoulders for our walk down the enclosed hall of our condo building. Partly for my own good, and partly to not disappoint Carol, I hobbled farther than I wanted while wondering with each step how I was going to get back. The afternoons were interchangeable with the mornings and, for that matter, so were the evenings until bed time when my routine of not sleeping continued.

Since I had not previously had a sleeping problem, I assumed mine was a transient one caused by my heart problems. In the hospital, while I used naps, I rationalized that my not sleeping much at night was a strength because it was caused by my spirit fighting to not give up control. I now realized whether or not this habit was a strength, it now was a weakness.

I had a great deal of time to think. I was so sorry to have been the cause of Carol's receiving the telephone call from the cardiologist. I missed my children and wished I could have prevented the shock of their almost losing me after they lost their mother so early in their lives. Carol became my voice to my world by providing updates on my status. I was happy to have my daughter, Hollie, visit from Seattle, but I slept for days afterwards. I loved talking to family and friends but had to strain to make my voice heard over the phone. I became so exhausted during telephone conversations that Carol started providing a warning near the ten minute mark. At 15 minutes, I would give the phone to her. I struggled to focus on anything for any length of time. My world had shrunk to one of survival and hope. But I had a world. Leaving the comfortable care of the hospital was a frightening, but necessary, step towards returning to an independent life style. The expression "no pain, no gain" used in athletics came to mind. The trick was to recognize beforehand whether an activity would help, or hurt, me. In an ethereal way this was, and is, really the challenge inherent in the title of this chapter: "Going Home Again."

CHAPTER 13. LESSONS LEARNED WHILE IN THE HOSPITAL

While many of my lessons learned may be applicable to all patients, my perspective was a heart patient whose cardiologist said, "Your problems were about as extreme as it gets." These words inspired me to write this book because if my program worked for such an extreme condition as mine, and it did, then it would work for almost any condition. If this message is important, and it is, then it almost had to be delivered by me since there are so few of us available to provide the first person perspective of rehabilitating after heart failure and the ensuing lung problems (estimated odds of one in a 100 million).

Mine is a message of hope. Hope because it is almost guaranteed that everybody else's problems will be less extreme than mine, and "Managing Your (my) Rehabilitation Program WELL," worked for me! It may be helpful to think of the acronym for WELL as Will Enthusiastically Love Life. Hope, according to thesaurus.com, represents "aspirations, desires, wishes, ambitions, goals, plans" (goals and plans will be discussed in detail later in this book) is powerful and, in the darkest hours, "hope" is often what separates those who will be successful from those who won't.

As the number one cause of death in the United States, there has been a great deal written about heart problems by well trained and highly skilled professionals. I am very appreciative of the medical professionals who did such wonderful things to enable me, with a little help, to go from life-to-death and back again to life; hence the name of the book "One Heart—Two Lives." This is not in any way to diminish their skills or dedication but rather to supplement their body of knowledge with the lessons learned from being a grateful recipient of these efforts.

Put in a lighter way, physicians' perspective is from looking down at patients in a hospital bed and wondering what the patients are feeling and thinking, and my patient's perspective is of looking up from the bed knowing what I think and feel and wondering what the physicians are thinking and feeling. The value of the different perspectives was proven to me when after years of asking questions of defendants who were sitting in what I described as the least comfortable seat in a deposition or court room---the witness chair-- I was called as a witness first in a deposition and then tool the long walk to the witness chair beside the judge's bench in a federal court room. When I put my hand on the Bible, I learned that my description of the lack of comfort in those chairs was an understatement. However the lessons I learned from those chairs helped me counsel clients on how to avoid those chairs and when unavoidable, taking the responsibility for the results. Similarly, I hope my taking responsibility for being a patient will be valuable to the medical community as well as former, current and future patients.

This is my attempt to share the many lessons I learned about survival, and life itself. My background has been included to assist readers' understanding of the perspective of the writer, as well as providing a summary of the settings in which the lessons were learned. I realize that there were people who genuinely tried to understand my feelings, which at the time I neither understood nor was able to vocalize, but which I believe were not unique to me. I am now sharing not only the physical problems, but also the emotions that are so important to our recoveries. Physicians can improve the physical structure but the mental/emotional ones, which I frequently refer to as attitude, are up to us; but are essential to "Managing Your Rehabilitation Program WELL." Physical efforts alone would not have been sufficient for me to overcome the odds which, when calculated cumulatively, were greater than a hundred million to one. It is my hope that others can learn from my experiences and not have to gamble on these odds.

The "Lessons Learned" sections are presented in the hope that others may learn from my experiences. This chapter contains the ones I learned while in the hospital. Many future chapters will conclude with a Lessons Learned section related to the lessons illustrated in that chapter so readers can understand how this patient learned these lessons. This method of demonstrating the reasons behind the lessons, and sometimes the immediate results, may make the lessons more relevant than just reading a list of them written by experts who may, or may not, have ever been heart patients. In some places the experiences have been supplemented by past experiences from the author's personal life, education, career or medical experiences. In each case the inclusion was to illustrate points. There are summaries of some medical issues to assist readers in becoming more knowledgeable about heart issues; be they potential, actual or former heart patients, family members, friends or caregivers. Medical issues are presented from a patient's perspective for the same reason. Please note that the intent was to alert readers to general concepts, not to replace the care of skilled, caring physicians.

In a strange way I was an ideal candidate to have these experiences and write this book. Don't get me wrong, I would not have volunteered. And to be sure, some of my stress was preventable, even though my parents' stress were passed down to me and were helpful career wise. And some were not, such as the three year plus struggle with cancer by my first wife, which did help to sensitize me to being a caregiver to a loved one. There were many other stress generating circumstances, like being a single parent of three children under ten years old while working a full time in a stressful job, the disaster of my house, and many more experiences. My background was presented to enable readers to learn from the things I did right, as well as the far too many things I did not, as well as to provide examples of my lessons learned.

At the time my heart stopped, I was taking what is generally thought of as "due care:" I did not smoke, my cholesterol was within acceptable limits, I was overweight but not obese, I exercised more than the amount prescribed by physicians and the national averages and I was blessed with great genes. I had annual physicals. In early 2006, a cardiologist said after a stress echo test, "Have a good life."

My exceptional circumstances of having taken, and taught, mathematics, management, industrial engineering, statistics, law and employment law, in addition to my practicing "people law" as Chief Employment Counsel for tens of thousands of employees, all contributed to helping me understand the physical, mental and emotional aspects of rehabilitating as well as the rights and duties of patients, professionals and volunteers; and my writing experience inspired me to share my perspective in the hopes others may benefit.

25 LESSONS LEARNED AS A PATIENT IN A HOSPITAL

When you are admitted to a hospital, your options become limited. But remember if the procedure works, or doesn't, regardless if the professional feels good, or bad: You must live with the results. You can delegate analysis and treatment, you can and should seek advice, counsel and treatments, but you cannot delegate the responsibility.

I learned this lesson years ago when I was admitted to the hospital for back spasms on a Friday. Over the weekend while I was strung up in traction, no physician appeared. On Monday an orthopedist entered my room and said in a sarcastic voice, "Who hooked you up like that. That is not doing you any good." I responded, "That other doctor in the green coat," to which he said, "That was no doctor as doctors only wear white coats." That wasted weekend in the hospital taught me a powerful lesson in who was ultimately responsible. Thinking "like a lawyer," I developed a standard question of, "This is important to me. Explain to me how this works and what I can do to make it more effective?" Learning this lesson sooner might have prevented a weekend of useless traction.

The mental/emotional side of the recovery is your job. When entering into the care of a physician, focus on maximizing the result and subsequently on recovering. As a patient in the hospital, plan to:

1. Be polite and cooperative. Everybody is trying to help you, so try to help them, like I did to the nurse from the rehabilitation center.

2. Don't make a veterinarian out of your doctor. Describe what you are feeling, for example, when I told the technician that the insulin shots made me feel queasy.

3. When possible, ask what alternatives are available to surgeries, treatments, and procedures, as my suggesting to the technician an alternative method to giving the insulin shots.

4. Ask the names of the medicines or injections and their

purposes. This will serve as a double check for the busy nurses and technicians, as well as alert you to the potential side effects.

5. Physical condition can affect attitude. A lesson I learned was that attitude can also affect our physical condition. Stay focused on getting well, as my walking when I really did not feel like it.

6. Don't sweat the small stuff, like the food, the channels on television, early morning tests, room temperatures or cold hands; this will distract you from focusing on getting well. For example, I did not complain about the early morning blood tests.

7. Get used to small hospital gowns and enjoy that someone else still cares what your posterior looks like, and enjoy the smiles as I did.

8. The top three ways to help your own recovery are attitude, attitude, and attitude! Studies indicate that it helps your recovery and there is no data that indicates it hinders it. Stack the deck in your favor. If you are positive, you will also tend to get quicker service.

9. It is sign of your recovery when you start thinking about the stresses your illness is placing on others, such as family, friends and support people. Be certain to express your appreciation to them like I did to the volunteer with the dog.

10. Use your time constructively: it will make it go faster, keep you from feeling sorry for yourself and improve your life after the hospital, like I did when I thought it might be my last day alive.

11. Don't ask, "why me?" Asking it will make you feel like a victim. Direct your focus on your recovery and later search for ways to prevent a recurrence.

12. A problem is only a problem until you have a plan; then it is a series of action items, like my getting ready for my surgeries.

13. Think about and visualize the wonders of your body and feel lucky to be alive like I tried to do before every surgery or procedure, such as the final one in the bathroom.

14. Try to help others with a smile and when possible, a kind word, like I was able to do by providing a legal opinion to Dr. W.

15. Remember as long as you are alive you have a chance to improve, which was why I was so thrilled to wake up after each surgery.

16. Rehabilitation starts almost immediately as muscle atrophy can start in as little as three days. Most post surgical problems occur because of inactivity: embrace it as I did for my walks.

17. It is your life. When you leave, the professionals will have another patient, but you will not have another life, so take responsibility for yourself like I did by reordering the sequence for the insulin shots.

18. Ask the hard questions like I did about the scheduling of my heart surgery.

19. Success and failure can be habits. Think of reasons why you can do something and not why you can't. The football coach Vince Lombardi said, "Show me a graceful loser and I'll show you a loser."

20. Focus on how you are going to handle positive results. If they happen, you will be ready and any worrying about negative ones will have been fruitless and unproductive; if they don't happen, there will be time to deal with the negative results. This worked for me on the Saturday before heart surgery that I thought might be my last day alive.

21. Your body is the key to your recovery. The treatments are meant to give your body the opportunity to heal itself; much like a bandage does not heal a wound but holds it closed, giving your body the opportunity to heal itself. A more personal example is my carotid and heart surgeries did not fix my irregular heart beat but did give my body the opportunity to heal itself; which it did.

22. Give your body the food it needs to heal, even when you don't like a particular serving.

23. Your body needs sleep. When you are awake your body burns energy. When you sleep, it can direct its energy to healing you.

24. Visualization and animation are wonderful tools, and psychologically help me as it did before each surgery.

25. Maintain your sense of humor. It is very difficult to complain when you are laughing. The visit by my friend Stan with the Junior Mints helped reduce the stress. As my wife used to say while fighting cancer, "It is not the troubles you have, but how you handle them that matters."

10 SUGGESTIONS FOR VISITORS TO PATIENTS IN HOSPITALS

1. First and foremost: Your presence is important and, at times, crucial. Please keep your visits short and often.

2. Please offer positive support through smiles, words, hugs and most importantly, attitude. Your attitude will influence a patient's attitude which will, in turn, influence his or her ability to recover.

3. You can start by taking care of yourself.

4. Help without being asked.

5. Talk to the adult patient like adults while remembering that medications may affect their ability to focus or communicate.

6. Talk about your life, family, friends, pets, plants, residence, job, bills, hobbies and any other interests you normally would discuss.

7. It comforts patients to know that their responsibilities such as jobs, bills, and residences are under control.

8. Support the professionals' efforts to help.

9. Help prevent the professionals from making mistakes by asking questions.

10. Please remember that the patient is still the same person, although they may act a little differently in the hospital.

5 THINGS TO BRING SOMEONE IN A HOSPITAL

1. Hope for tomorrow through a smile and an encouraging word.

2. A story about something from the patient's past that hopefully will also be in their future.

3. Be careful about bringing food. The patient may be on a particular type of diet or may have temporary chewing, swallowing or digesting problems.

4. Reading material even though the patient may not be able to concentrate due to their condition or medications.

5. Photographs are great especially if there is available shelf space within a line of vision.

STAY RELEASED

Studies show that one in five Medicare beneficiaries return to the hospital within 30 days of their release (Medicare Payment Advisory Commission). For heart patients, besides the risk of a recurrence of the same problem, there is the risk of related problems, such as Post Traumatic Stress Disorder (PTSD) where of an estimated 1.4 million patients discharged from hospitals after heart attacks or other acute coronary events, an estimated 168,000 will develop PTSD (chapter 32).

CHAPTER 14. RELEARNING TO BREATHE, EAT AND SLEEP

<u>Monday</u>: I woke at home with thoughts that "It was the best of times, it was the worst of times," parroting the eloquent opening line from *The Tale of Two Cities* (Charles Dickens 1812-1870). It felt great, and scary, to be home again. Great because it meant I had progressed to the point of being capable of being released. Scary my dependency on a team of trained, dedicated healthcare professionals, was ending. Now there was only my wife, Carol, whose caring was handicapped by her lack of training and time as she still had a stressful, full time job, and me. Partially to relieve her, and partially through my desire to function more independently, I wanted to assume more responsibility for myself. However, besides not being physically able, I would learn just how unready I was psychologically. Coming home did give me a feeling that the professionals thought my need for help had decreased, although the reality was that it freed them up for new patients by shifting my dependency to Carol.

Capability wise, I should have still been in the hospital. The hospital had taken full responsibility for my physical condition, including helping me correct my heart's rhythm, disposal of waste, and whatever else I needed except, of course, a gown that closed in the back. When they determined that I no longer needed monitoring 24/7 to physically survive, they released me. I am extremely grateful for my hospital experience. Simply put, they did everything physically necessary to help me be recalled to life. But as with all good things, it had to end. As an aside, I can't imagine how difficult it must be for longer term hospital patients to have to adjust to leaving an environment where each day increases their dependency.

Being released from the hospital felt great, but it always was only a preliminary objective. Being at home showed me how far I still had to go to accomplish my longer term objective of living independently. Watching Carol trying to decide what I needed next, from what I would wear to what I would eat, brought immense sadness. I did not like what I was doing to her. I was no more independent than I had been in the hospital. Fortunately my "thinking" power was somewhere between the haze of the anesthetic and normal, so many of these thoughts were still being formulated. Mornings began with Carol helping me get out of bed, dressing me in the clothes she had just purchased for their ease in putting them on, helping me walk to the couch in the living room and sitting down. Then while I sat still, Carol hustled to adjust the pillows on the couch and place the foot stool in just the right position to support my left leg to reduce the swelling. Sitting on the stool, Carol strained to pull up my medical sock on my left leg that was swollen from the surgery where the vein used for my bypass was removed. There was no chance that I could do it myself, no matter how important it was, and it was very important. I strained to even provide the necessary resistance with my leg. Carol provided me with a warm jacket, since after my surgeries I tended to get chilled much quicker than I used to. Then she turned on the television, cooked and served breakfast; all before she got dressed and started her work as a corporate secretary.

In the hospital, I had started to take some responsibility for myself with actions like questioning the purpose and timing of the tests and injections. To make light of my number one fear, that of returning to the cardiac ward, I thought of it as "not greeting my visitors horizontally." Now I was at a cross roads of doing only the physical activities that I was completely comfortable with, which were very few, or to risk doing activities outside my comfort zone in order to decrease my long term dependence on others. This battle between short term comfort and long term independence would influence almost every movement. My analytical side, or according to neurologists, the left side of my brain, said "We are lucky. Our physicians said we have no restrictions." The debate was on. My emotional or right side of my brain said "Did you ask?"

Left side, "No, but neither did you." Right side, "I am emotional. I did not ask because I was afraid of a negative answer. But you are supposed to be factual and not afraid of the truth."

Left side, "Don't you start that crap: The physicians would have indicated restrictions, if there were any, and they did not; so there aren't any." Right side, "Yeah, right, they also said during your annual physical last year that you were fine. How did that work out?"

Left side, "I know. I was there too. But we really have no choice. So this time we will have to monitor ourselves." Right side, "How do you plan to do that Mr. Analytical?"

Left side, "Well, Mr. Emotional, we will have to learn that as we go." Right side, "Nice idea but how do you intend to do that?"

Left side, "I will ask before engaging in any activity whether it will help, or hurt, me." The right side said, "Sort of the ultimate gamble: will we learn enough before the lessons harm us."

The left side, "I am not thrilled with this approach, but without it we have no hope."

So I would push activities that provided the best chances of leading to independence and hope that by monitoring them I could prevent a relapse. My new mantra was for each activity to ask: help or hurt? I had to start with the most basic survival needs: the physiological ones of air, water, food, and sleep. All other needs were secondary. The Texas Heart Institute identified a similar list of concerns for post surgical heart patients of "sleep problems, not feeling hungry, feeling very tired, not caring about things that used to be important to you, and having a low self esteem." (texasheartinstitute.org). Here was my approach:

Medicines: Physicians could provide me a physiological framework but it was my responsibility to follow their guidance. Besides regular checkups, this included taking my prescriptions, which were:

-- A calcium channel blocker to improve blood flow,

-- A beta-blocker to improve circulation,

-- A "water" pill to prevent my body from absorbing too much salt,

-- A pill to block the production of cholesterol,

-- An aspirin, in my case a "baby" one, as an anti-inflammatory,

-- With the approval of physicians, I added omega 3 to lower triglycerides, a multiple vitamin, and vitamins C and B12.

My being grateful that there were pills that could improve my life quickly overcame any feelings of inadequacy at needing daily pills, which I tended to call "vitamins" as I took them first thing every morning with breakfast.

Air: Our most basic need to live is to breathe; and less obvious, is that to live better requires that we breathe better. My challenge was to improve my breathing by taking deeper breaths, by breathing through my diaphragm to re-open my lungs and regain the capacity lost during heart surgery. The only tool I had was the Voldyne. All I had to do was blow a ball up a few inches. When my first couple of blows did not move the ball, like a good pin ball machine player I banged my hand on the side of tube: still no movement. When turned upside down, the ball moved. So it was not broken: I was. I had to blow harder. I tried to follow the instructions and blow ten times, three times a day. My routine became having the ball ignore me on my first blow as I warmed up. Taking deeper breaths and blowing harder may have moved it a tad on my second and third attempts. Each failure increased my determination, as I am my father's son, and increased my willingness to risk breaking my staples and stitches by blowing too hard. I kept blowing until the ball moved about half way up the tube. My chest ached but did not break open. During my sixth attempt sweat moistened my hair, or as my wife would say, "perspiration." During my eighth attempt, the sweat ran into my eyes. On the ninth attempt, which proved to be my best, the ball moved past the half-way mark. The tenth attempt was a relief blow with no real chance of success. I remembered my friend F.X.O. saying that all folks like a complete story, which he compared to a circle. If they only had part of the story, or circle, they would complete it with what they thought fit. I decided that "completing the circle" required that I "ring the bell," so three times a day for weeks I tried harder to reopen my lungs.

I was learning a great deal about breathing, such as a simple test for the important concept of using my diaphragm was when drawing air in, my stomach should contract, and when letting it out, my stomach should expand. Since our bodies need the oxygen supplied by our lungs in order to do anything from digesting food to moving, declining capacity will reduce all our bodies' ability to perform vital functions.

The process to reduce lung capacity was easy: just do nothing. To accelerate the decrease, just smoke. The process to increase the capacity was long, hard, painful and at this point required the mastering of the Voldyne. I was learning to appreciate some of the things people with permanent restrictions experience and to understand that many people fall asleep on airplanes because of the reduced supply of oxygen.

Water and Fluids: Lack of water can lead to "dehydration," which drains energy and make us tired. We lose it through breath, perspiration, urine and bowel movements, which is accelerated by exercise, hot, humid weather, altitude and illness or other health issues (mayoclinic.com). The Institute of Medicine provides that, on the average, men should drink 3 liters or 13 cups of water a day and women 2.2 liters, or 9 cups daily. Both are equivalent to the health care professionals recommendations of "drink 8 glasses of 8 ounces."

Fortunately I was permitted to continue to enjoy the smell, taste, and the way coffee made me feel. There was a familiarity with the coffee in those decorative mugs that fit my hand so well. The usual effect in the morning helped snap me out of morning hazes and the lingering effects of the anesthetic, which also greatly reduced my body's ability to produce adrenaline. Everything was so complicated, like drinking more water and coffee meant more painful trips to the bathroom.

Food: I grew up hearing about my mother's voice saying, "Take what you can eat, and eat what you take," a habit that was challenged by the oysters stews on Friday nights because my father's pay check would not clear the bank until Monday.

In the hospital there was so much going on that food was not a priority. At home, Carol's first meal alerted my senses. It was the simple meal many newlywed women prepared, besides spaghetti, of ham, scrambled eggs, potatoes and toast, yet the colors and smells stimulated my hunger. Hunger that was satisfied in just a couple of bites. I tried to finish because I did not want to disappoint Carol or my own childhood expectations. However, my surgery had so reduced my ability to digest any more or, for that matter, to handle the stress of even this mild conflict. As my eyes filled, I said with a shaky voice, "Carol, I cannot eat any more." She responded, "That's all right, just eating what you can is fine." I said, "But I don't want to waste food. Next time don't make as much." She said, "Food is important for your recovery." Having an objective voice is important.

Eating gives the body the nutrients it needs to recover. Eating the right foods, that is. Carol grew up on a farm where vegetables were the mainstay of her family's meals. I grew up in a suburb where my German descent father was known to say he could eat roast beef and mashed potatoes every night with, maybe, a small portion of green beans. The highlight of Sunday brunch at Carol's was scrambled eggs: at my house it was spreading butter on cinnamon buns and crumb cakes. Carol knew where to find the freshest vegetables: I knew where to find the best donuts. Carol was still standing: I had to change.

From the tons of material available on eating healthy, we loosely followed the guidelines from the American Heart Association (AHA). In general at least twice a week we replaced red meats with oily fish, like salmon and chicken, and ate a lot of fruits and vegetables. We did find the eat "less than" group of foods difficult to measure, like less salt, as it tends to increase the very blood pressure I was taking pills to reduce, and the less than 7% of calories coming from saturated fats; less than 1% of calories from Tran's fats; less than 300 mg of dietary cholesterol a day (Cleveland clinic.org). There were times when I found solace by repeating that "I was going to eat to live, rather than live to eat."

The key is that somehow, some way, every patient will improve when they get access to a balanced diet. Achieving this is a great way for supporters to contribute, but they should be aware of potential appetite reductions and a preference for the forbidden foods. It felt funny, in an odd way, that after years of trying to eat less I was now trying to eat more. As time passed, I began to appreciate the natural spices and flavors of my new diet. It just took time.

Sleep: When I was working I took pride in getting by on less than eight hours of sleep per night, so I may have been one of the 40 million people that do not get enough sleep (Center for Disease Control). In the hospital I learned that sleep was when my body could use its energies towards healing itself.

Insomnia comes in various forms. Some people have trouble falling asleep, some in waking up in the middle of the night and going back to sleep, and others in waking up too early (sleepfoundation). Studies show that 30% of American adults have some symptoms and 10% have chronic insomnia, which is generally defined as having difficulty sleeping at least three times a week for a month or more. Chronic insomnia sufferers may also feel tired, cranky or foggy-headed during the day, and can have an increased risk for other conditions, including heart disease, diabetes and depression (Mayo Clinic).

My sleeping problems in the hospital were consistent with "transient" insomnia, which is when someone occasionally experiences a few nights of tossing and turning. This type of insomnia can be caused by medical conditions, such as depression, sleep apnea, arthritis, chronic pain and heart failure, which I thought caused mine. I reluctantly started a prescription for a sleeping pill that indicated a 6-8 hours duration. Some reports confirm that sleeping pills may not last the listed duration (Consumer Reports, 2012), and I woke after 2-3 hours. I had very little of the potential side effects of daytime drowsiness, memory or balance problems, while women and individuals over age 65 years of age are more likely to have adverse reactions because they tend to have slower metabolisms (Scripps Clinic Family Sleep Center).

The market for sleeping pills is huge (sixty million prescriptions written in 2010) and half of the 19,487 trips to Emergency Rooms in 2010 were by individuals who had also taken sleeping pills along with narcotic pain relievers and other medications to treat anxiety and insomnia (Substance Abuse and Mental Health Services Administration). Sleeping pills "are not an alternative to taking a look at your life and figuring out why you're having a sleeping problem," said a past president of the American College of Physicians (Andrea Petersen, Wall Street Journal, July 19, 2011).

Again the opening sentence of *The Tale of Two Cities* so eloquently expressed my exiting January: "it was the spring of hope, it was the winter of despair" and how I managed my rehabilitation program would determine whether "we had everything before us, we had nothing before us."

Lessons Learned:

1. Take responsibility for the procedures for your recovery, such as the appropriate amounts of air, fluids, food, and sleep.

2. Heart problems can, and must, be viewed as a learning experience for both the things to do as well as those to avoid since whatever caused the problem may well cause it again.

CHAPTER 15. FEBRUARY: A FORMAL REHABILITATION PROGRAM

For me February began with the question: Would a formal (conventional, approved, validated) rehabilitation (bring someone to a healthy condition) program (a plan of things that are done to achieve a specific result), meaning one run by professional (a person who earns their living from a specific activity) nurses (assists individuals in activities contributing to health or its recovery), be worth my time? Once the definitions of the terms are spelled out, it is difficult see how a thinking person could question whether such a program could be helpful. However, my energy levels were so limited that I was reluctant to spent them on group activities because of my experiences with groups as a student, professor and attorney, were, to be kind, not always positive and, to be blunter, far too often a waste of time and energies, as the tendencies always seemed to be for the group to drift off the relevant topics. I liked interactions with people but group activities were a different matter.

From the nurse's hospital visit I did not understand the structure of the "formal" rehabilitation program, where I added the word "formal" to differentiate these structured activities controlled by professionals from my unstructured ones. I was skeptical but I decided to at least try every available resource before deciding whether to participate. Besides, I knew my method of trying to determine beforehand whether each activity would "help or hurt" me was doomed to failure because I could never answer it: so every activity became a gamble.

While I was in the hospital there was no paradox as the professionals made the decisions. At home the "professional" was me. Slowly, carefully, day-by-day, step-by-step, I tried this laborious, uncertain method to add any new movements: what a stress generator. This time was different from my previous training in pushing myself to the limit and then doing a little more. This time the risks were not to my skin, muscles, bones or ligaments; they could all be repaired. The real risks were twofold: one, to my heart which might not be repairable; two, to my fragile confidence. My attempts to monitor my heart rate were crude and ineffective since activities always make your heart beat faster.

So the question was whether the formal program would help me in learning to "Manage Your (my) Rehabilitation Program WELL?"

Nurse L, who ran the formal rehabilitation program, was part of the cardiology department, so I figured she must know what she was doing. My lack of progress at home and my resolution to do all that I could to return to a full, independent life caused me to consider the program.

My drive to the clinic was easy: entering it was not. I had entered it frequently in my first life but this time was different. I approached the front doors at a pace that would have embarrassed a person with a walker. I slowed this pace down even further when I realized this was my first visit of my second life. The newspaper stand on my left still declared headlines about national matters that used to interest me. The pharmacy on my right never was interesting. The automatic glass doors slid open, exposing the lobby I never really noticed before as I walked to the elevators on my left. Instinctively, I glanced at my watch during the elevator ride to the third floor. I got chills. My memory was right. If my heart had not stopped in the Cardiology Department, but in the elevator on my way out of the clinic, the slowness of the elevator would have virtual guaranteed my suffering brain damage or worse. I shakily shuffled off onto the third floor and followed the arrow pointing left to the Cardiology Department. On my sixth step, the wall on my left opened into a waiting room half full of people. Scanning the waiting room showed eyes peering over the tops of magazines, as mine used to do, looking for signs of what was wrong with the new arrival. The fear levels in the eyes differentiated the patients from the people accompanying them. Some of them would be leaving breathing a sigh of relief; some hoping the next test would be better; some praying to receive a miracle. Unbeknownst to one pair of eyes, the back cover of the magazine being held proclaimed another category of hope: How to have a Better Sex Life. I looked to the nurses' station to my right where the nurses were talking about last night's dates. I started hoping the door marked Cardiac Rehabilitation was locked: it wasn't.

PHYSICAL REHABILITATION PROGRAM: I was greeted by a short, thin lady dressed in the traditional nurse's outfit, who I recognized as nurse L. She introduced me to nurse J., another nurse whose warm smile welcomed me to the program. These two were to be my rehab team and so much more.

My first glances around the room humbled me. It wasn't the room: it was bright, open with two walls of windows, and reasonably cheerful. It wasn't the equipment: the three treadmills straight ahead, the two stationary bikes to the right and the arm strength machines all resembled those found in gyms. It wasn't the chairs: they were fine. It was the other patients: they looked so feeble. On the left treadmill a man was trying to walk as close to zero miles an hour as humanly possible. In the middle, one a woman was eyeing the six inch step up as if it was six feet. I don't belong in this group, I thought, I belong in the category advertised on the magazine cover as only a couple of hours ago I had snuck peaks at Carol emerging from the shower and felt a stirring. I quickly decided that I would not be here if I did not belong, so get over it and just become the best student.

L. led me to the chairs under the window to my left, where she explained that at every visit I would be fitted with a monitoring harness with a constant feed to individual computer screens in the center portion of the room. Vitals related to my heart would be continually taken and compared to my records. Classes were kept small, typically between 3-4 people, and met twice a week for approximately an hour. Each time I was to perform on each type of machine. Their primary goals for me were compatible with mine: gradually increasing my exercise in a controlled environment while learning to monitor myself. I liked the program and signed up for Tuesday and Thursday classes.

Nurse L. fitted me with a harness, a nice word for an electronic device to monitor my heart, which I thought of as a continuous EKG with the instructions to relax: nice idea, wrong patient. She sent me to the middle tread mill where I now understood the other patient's having trouble stepping up. My knuckles grasping the handles turned white. Once a treadmill starts, there is no such thing as one foot on and one foot off. I was off with the same wobbly, stiff kneed, disjointed set of movements as a child learning to walk. Over the weeks my confidence increased so much that I started to create story lines for the folks in the red tile roofs visible through the floor-to-ceiling glass windows.

My next stop was the stationary bikes. Unlike the treadmill there was a gauge to measure my rate of peddling. My tendency, a gentle word for determination, was to try and peddle at exactly the specified rate. As I became more comfortable, I would look out the windows across the room and visualize hiking up the sides of the Santa Ynez Mountains.

My final stop was the toughest for me; the hand crank machine on the table adjacent to the door. The procedure was simple enough: the resistance was set before I grasped the handle and turned the wheel a specified number of revolutions per minute.

I noticed that patients self-divided into two groups: those who were creative in finding reasons to attend, and those who were equally as creative in finding reasons to be absent. Some reasons, such as going shopping or being tired, may be valid for some activities but were highly questionable for rehab. Day-by-day the encouragement and security of being monitored was helping me to achieve my objective of developing a method for monitoring myself.

One day as a new class mate's treadmill was spinning much faster than mine, I broke my typical silent routine by asking this younger, healthier looking stranger, "What was your surgery?"

"I did not have surgery," he responded.

Confused, I asked "Then why are you here?"

"To try to strengthen my heart. After my surgery sixteen years ago, I felt so good that I did not follow their directions to exercise. Now I have another problem but the doctors tell me my heart muscles are too weak for surgery."

"What are you going to do?"

"All I can do is attend rehab and hope." In another class, I overheard him telling L. that he had kayaked in the Pacific at Morro Bay. This small waterfront town is known as the Gibraltar of the Pacific, because of the distinguishing rock that dominates the large harbor. The configuration of the harbor causes a huge volume of water to funnel past the narrow channel by the rock with the changing of the tides. The tide helped him paddle his kayak out passed the rock. But when he tried to return against the tide, he felt chest pains as he was being swept farther out to sea. "The tide was winning," he said, "I was going out to sea without a cell phone, anyone to wave to, and no one to yell to except the sea gulls sitting on the buoy that I was just able to grab." He continued, "I could feel the strain on my heart as the tide pulled my kayak. I got lucky when someone sent help." The pain in his voice was a powerful incentive for taking the steps to avoid having this type of experience in my future.

Subsequently, I learned that he was in the majority: the statistics for heart patients continuing to exercise were not encouraging. A study of the participation rate for cardiac rehab exercise programs showed that within six months of their heart surgeries only 50% of the former heart patients would still be exercising. Within 12 to 18 months the percentage drops to 30%, which is about the national average for everyone to exercise. In other words, within a year to a year and a half most post surgical heart patients will return to the exercise levels they had while they were developing heart disease. While these percentages are estimates they are consistent with another study that found only 22% of adults in the U.S. exercise 5 times week for at least 30 minutes per time.

REHABILITATION LECTURES: I reluctantly entered the room where the lecture part of the rehabilitation program was being held once a week for two hours. As with the exercise program, I decided to try a lecture or two and stop if I did not like them. I never missed a lecture. Actually, they were a combination of lecture and interactive exchanges including excellent written materials. The lectures were:
1. Your Heart and how it Works,
2. Risk Factors and Coronary Artery Disease,
3. Diet: Cooking and Eating Out,
4. Healthy Diet: the Right Choices,
5. Exercise,
6. Cardiac Blues,
7. Stress Reduction, and
8. Lifestyles.
I roughly divided the lectures into four groupings as follows;

A. General information, or lectures number 1 and 2, which provided an understanding of how our hearts work with an emphasis on the inter-relationships of the various parts and problems that can occur.

B. The physical aspects, or lectures number 3, 4 and 5, which provided guidance on how to improve our diets and exercise and their inter-relationships.

C. The mental aspects, or lectures 6 and 7, which provided guidance on handling the frustrations and fears that frequently follow heart surgery, as well as ways to reduce stress.

D. Lifestyles, or lecture 8, which provided guidance on integrating the other suggestions into a satisfying lifestyle.

I was particularly interested in the Cardiac Blues lecture on managing stress, which was given by Mr. B., a PhD psychologist. The doctor's voice conveyed his pain, and fear, as he discussed his family's history of heart disease, which had inspired him to study the importance of relationships in reducing stress. He urged us to cherish and nurture our relationships by making time for our love ones while we handle our heart problems. I felt his pain as he told us that his father kept promising to take him fishing but never did before his time ran out. I was moved and related that when my father retired, he bought two fishing poles with the intent of fishing and golfing with me. We never fished but I still treasure the one time we golfed and he talked about reducing his swing to keep the golf ball on the fairway after having had "other" experiences during his once a year golf outing at the DuPont Country Club. While vowing to do better with my sons and daughter, like the doctor, I knew in order to lead a healthier life; I had to learn how to manage the stresses that had been a major contributor to my problems. All too soon after his lecture, the doctor lost his battle with stress and passed away from heart disease. This hit me hard: what chance did I have of managing my stress if my ten year younger expert on stress died from his? I searched for a way to break my feelings of helplessness. Finally, my subconscious came through. My program was the way to continue to be a survivor!

The statistics presented in the Lifestyle Lecture were troubling. Managing four lifestyle characteristics (smoking, weight, diet and exercise) was identified as being important in reducing heart disease. A survey of adults in the United States showed that:

-Not smoking was practiced by 75% of the folks,

-Keeping weight between 18.5 to 25 on the Body Mass Index (BMI) was practiced by 40%,

-Maintaining a diet of at least 5 fruits and vegetables per day was observed by 23%,

-Exercising at least 5 times a week for at least 30 minutes per time was practiced by 23%,

-Consistently achieving all of the above 4 goals was practiced by only 3%.

These numbers showed me that 97% of adults are not doing all that they can reduce potential heart disease. I had always felt pretty good about myself since I had not smoked and exercised the designated amount. But this study showed me that I still needed to work on eating 5 fruits and vegetables and keeping my weight within the designated BMI range.

The formal rehabilitation program was terrific. Day-to-day, movement-by-movement, encouragement-by-encouragement, the nurses helped me find a way to answer "will it help or hurt me?" Building my confidence to be able to monitor myself so I could stop before I got into too much trouble was the missing key.

The formal rehabilitation program greatly helped me to learn, in a controlled environment, at least some of the movements that would help, not hurt, me, and to be able to tell the difference, as well as to sensitize me to how our bodies work. The combination of the physical and lecture parts were very valuable in my learning to "Manage Your (my) Rehabilitation Program WELL," as well as "Will Enthusiastically Love Life.

Lessons Learned:

1.Physicians can assist us to be physically able to pursue an active lifestyle, which is necessary but in itself, the next steps are security (safety), social (relationships), and esteem (a feeling of personal worth).

2.There is help available for heart patients, such as the formal rehab program, and the largest peer-to-peer organization n the world for heart patients, Mended Hearts, as well as the American Heart Association.

2. " Managing Your (my) Rehabilitation Program WELL would be worth whatever time and energy required: period!

CHAPTER 16. MARCH: FAMILY MONTH

Just seeing March at the top of the calendar always spread my lips into a wide smile. As a child it meant birthday month, first mine and two days later my brother's, as I blissfully ignored my father's being the first one of the month. After I became a father, and we lived in the northeast, March signified the beginning of the end of the fun of building snow men with my children until the sun caused my wing tip shoes to disappear into the ankle high slush on my way to work. As the snow decreased, and the ages of my children increased, snow again played a role in family fun. This time it was on the slopes of the Wasatch Mountains in Park City, Utah. What great days we had skiing and boarding the miles long trails from 9,250 feet altitude down to town level of 7,000 feet, followed by evenings in the hot tube exchanging our mountain versions of fish stories before dinner over March Madness. I looked forward to those weeks all year, which was especially true this year. Shortly after I thought surgery had cured my physical problems , I started planning to see my children in March.

Planning had always been important to me (discussed in detail later in this book). Even heart patients have thoughts, feelings and needs, which for me meant a need to be able to use planning as a spirit lifting technique as I waited for the sun to break through the endless nights.

I understood the reluctance of my cardiologist, or any professional, to provide a definite schedule for an indefinite process. In my legal practice those same reasons prevented my co-counsels from providing schedules for our litigation. So I used my expertise to create "tentative" schedules which, once drafted, my co-counsel always agreed since the modifier "tentative" provided for the unexpected. My cardiologist, with that same type of expertise, modifier, refused to respond to my tentative recovery schedule with even a risk free "we'll see," or "it depends." He remained silent. But since he did not say "no" I interpreted his silence the same way indicated by the lyrics from the song the "Sounds of Silence," "The vision that was planted in my brain, Still remains, Within the sounds of silence" (Simon and Garfunkel). My "tentative" schedule for Park City survived his silences.

Why March? March had always symbolized a "new beginning," as my father was born on the 6th; my first wife, Anne, on the 17th, my brother Barry on the 30th, friends Mike, Bob, Norm and JG, between the 23rd and the 31st, and my "original" birth date was the 28th.

Why Park City? My business travels caused me to fly into nearby Salt Lake City. The sun coming up over the beautiful Wasatch Mountains would highlight my drive to the huge, as in thousands of acres, facility spread up the side of a mountain so a detonation (a violent expansion of energy) or deflagration (a rapid burning),(a distinction that I learned while winning the largest case in the history of OSHA) would be funneled away from other people or places. This facility was ironically named the Bacchus Works after the Greek and Roman god of wine and revelry, since it was the only facility in the United States that manufactured solid fuel rocket motors for outer space, and the only one in the world that made first Poseidon, and then Trident, missiles that could be launched from submarines. That this was a key factor President Reagan used to cause the Soviets to agree to end the Cold War was indicated by the Soviets selecting , pursuant to this treaty, only the Bacchus Works, to construct a "demilitarized" zone in the middle of the facility, manned by their sixty "advisors," where they could inspect all our materials and products. My Top Secret security clearance was needed to handle some of the billion dollar legal issues while re-organizing the six thousand jobs and protecting our national security.

To escape these stresses, in the early evenings I would longingly wonder what it would be like to ski down the majestic, snow capped, mountains. Even though I could not ski, one Saturday morning I "escaped" the stresses by making the short drive up Route 80 to Park

City. The stresses of the modern world literally evaporated as I entered the historic district of this former silver mining town nestled in between majestic mountains. Shortly thereafter I found the Park Hotel and, at least for a few weeks in March, it has become the place for our family vacation. Every January, including this one, I start planning on seeing my children while staying in that quaint, small, European style hotel, which is known as the "blue building on Main Street with the friendly staff."

Why a family vacation? The short reason is that I love them. The longer one is that they will come if there is some fun activity. When my children were young our vacations were centered on the beach, particularly Ocean City, Maryland. As they all too quickly grew and learned how to ski or board, and my skiing progressed from my learning that strapping two straight boards on my feet would prevent my ever turning, our family vacations shifted to Park City. Over the years I developed three (would you expect anything less from a math major?) rules for each day: Have fun, learn a little bit and be able to ski again tomorrow. Each morning, after repeating the rules, we took the Town Lift to the top of the mountain where, after pausing to give thanks to the power that created these indescribably beautiful mountains and for permitting me to be able to share them. As the years passed I slowly shifted from being a stick man to "feeling" the mountain.

When this March arrived, I was full of confidence. In my formal rehab program I had increased the times on the treadmill, bike and arm machine, so I assumed I was progressing according to my tentative schedule and was not worried when the nurturing rehab nurse said the seven simple words, "it is time for a chest x-ray."

That is, until I learned that the x-ray showed that I was slowly suffocating myself. "Suffocating" because with each breath my body was taking, it became more difficult for my lungs to expand. I would learn that my defying the odds continued as I was one of the approximately 25% of patients who during open heart surgery lose the small amount of lubricant from the side walls of their lungs. Most lost it from the left side; I lost the right side. Most people's bodies reproduce it; mine did not. Without this lubricant, the expanding and contracting of my lungs caused a friction that my body detected as a problem and rushed so much fluid to my chest cavity that my body could not dispose of it. The growing volume shrunk the space needed for the next lung expansion so I was, in effect, slowly suffocating myself with the same technique used by boa constrictors to suffocate their victims. This must have been the reason why the Voldyne was so difficult. This was crushing news. I was thrilled to have been in the tiny statistical minority that survive their heart stopping, but I knew that continually betting against the averages was like repeatedly betting on filling an inside straight in poker: a guaranteed loser.

On a Friday passing through the sliding glass doors into the hospital, the same hospital where my last entrance had been on a gurney, so affected my breathing that I had to force deep breaths and repeat that this was for an "outpatient procedure." Outpatient as in this patient was walking out afterwards. We, Carol and I, went as directed, through the swinging doors on the left to a hallway with a waiting room on our left and, when I looked in the procedure room on our right, all I saw was a short, rotund, bearded man wearing a Hawaiian shirt. As I turned to leave, a voice said, "Are you Mr. Zepke?" I slowly turned looking for the speaker but the only person there was the Hawaiian shirt guy. How did he know my name? "Are you Mr. Zepke," he repeated. "I am your pulmonologist." My thoughts were "You might be 'a' pulmonologist, but you're not going to be 'my' pulmonologist." My mind raced: How can I gracefully get out of here. Should I deny being Mr. Zepke or simply leave?

Carol eliminated my dilemma when she broke the silence with, "Yes he is."

The Hawaiian shirt continued, "Please excuse my dress. Fridays are casual days." His smile and demeanor were reassuring and, in the theme of "beggars can't be choosy," I stripped to my waist, sat on the side of an examination table, placed my elbows on a metal cart and leaned forward with my elbows on the cart. He said, "A tube will be inserted into your back, through your ribs into your chest. The fluid in your chest will drain through the tube into a bottle placed behind you."

The visualization of the tube sliding in my back made me feel lightheaded. I froze, afraid to move since the table and cart were on wheels that were not locked. When I felt a marker drawing a circle in the middle of my back, I visualized a knife tracing the lines and felt any movement could cause the knife to cut more than intended. He made the cut and inserted the tube while I focused on Carol. At what seemed like an hour later, but probably was only a matter of minutes, the doctor's voice intruded on my efforts to stop my dizziness, with the words, "This bottle is full." My thoughts of, "we are finished," lasted only until his request to the nurse of "Please hand me another bottle." When he finally said, "The procedure is over," and removed the tube from my back, I asked what I thought was an easy question, "Did you get it all?" He responded, "I am not certain if I got it all, but I have found that taking more than two liters creates the potential for serious side effects." I was stunned. Did he really mean two liters? I searched for a way to visualize two liters, such as trying to stuff a two-liter bottle of soda into my chest. My mind raced: wasn't two litters equal to 66 ounces or 2.1 quarts? I am not that big.

The doctor continued, "Do you want to look at the fluid?"

"No thanks," I said wondering if he was serious. What I wanted was to get the heck out of there. As I stood up and put on my shirt, the power of suggestion got the best of me and I stole a glance at the bottle: serious mistake. The bottle was full of a reddish brown fluid. Now I would forever visualize this nasty looking stuff as being in my chest. However, with my first full inhaling I literally could feel the oxygen flowing through my chest, arms, legs and down to my toes. I stood a little taller, walked a little faster and looked at Carol a little differently as we strolled back through the lobby.

The doctor also prescribed an anti-inflammatory drug to slow my body from sending fluid and give it a chance to heal itself. Being able to take deeper breaths gave me so much confidence that I resumed planning my trip to Park City. My plans, however, for my activities had shifted from skiing to walking around this former mining town nestled at 7,000 feet in the mountains of Utah. I found a ray of hope from the good omen that March 17th, my scheduled departure date, was also my children's deceased mother's birthday. Besides celebrating her birthday, I also traditionally joined the Irish celebration of St. Patrick's Day in honor of my paternal Irish grandmother Brady.

For weeks Carol advised me to directly ask my cardiologist, repeatedly saying, "A difference between men and women is that men tend to talk around something, while women ask directly." When I finally asked directly, the male cardiologist gave no opinion. Instead he referred me back to the pulmonologist, where I was so confident of the results of our appointment on March 19th to discuss my next chest x-rays, that I moved my plane ticket back to March 21st. On the 19th, my hopes were lifted when the nurse, when taking my vitals, said, "You must be an athlete because your heart rate is so low." I entered a lab with a small bounce in my step until I saw the glass phone booth sized apparatus in the middle of the lab. "What the heck is that for?" I asked. Since my surgery, I had become slightly claustrophobic. The technician said it was to measure my breathing under controlled situations. I entered the booth and breathed into a clear plastic mask.

To learn the test results that afternoon, Carol and I were led into a small, narrow office where the pulmonologist so dwarfed the desk that he looked like a parent sitting in his child's desk on parents' night at a grammar school. He distractedly said to take a seat, and continued to frown as his hand flew over the keys of a calculator. I noticed a diploma on the wall, and asked, "Do you have a Ph.D. in Chemistry?"

"Yes," he responded. "After earning it, I decided I could better help people if I went to medical school. My research shows Park City is approximately 7,000 feet altitude. Is this trip important to you?"

"Yes," I said. "I really need to see my children."

His forehead wrinkled as he said, "I am not married and do not have any children, but I understand how important this might be to you." He turned back to his desk and started furiously writing. He winced as he handed me a prescription with the words, "You will have to have this prescription for portable oxygen filled in Park City." "Whoa," I stammered, "Portable oxygen?"

"Yes. As we go higher in altitude, the air becomes thinner and at an altitude of about 7,000 feet, the test projected your oxygen utilization rate as 58%. You will need to arrange for an oxygen source for 24/7."

I gasped. My thoughts raced back to the hospital when my utilization rate was "only" 91%, I was given oxygen. The doctor never said, and I was too scared to ask, what would happen at 58%, but we both knew. Any interruption in oxygen, even while showering, eating, sleeping or walking the steep streets, would be instantly fatal! The condition where the body is denied sufficient oxygen to supply body tissues is "hypobaric hypoxia" and is most common in air flights (myheartsisters.org).

The doctor handed me another prescription with the words, "This one is for a three- hour container of portable oxygen for the flight as the air pressure in airplanes is set to the pressure at 10,000 feet altitude, which is why at this altitude private pilots are advised to use oxygen. The thin oxygen may partially explain why people frequently fall asleep on flights." Had I heard him right: the portable oxygen would only last three hours? Was I betting my life that the plane would not have to sit on the runway? I was touched and appreciative of the doctor's efforts but now faced a dilemma: should I risk it all to see my children now, or delay my trip and trust that I would recover and spend quality time with them in the future?

My children understood, perhaps better than I did, that "Managing Your (my) Rehabilitation Program WELL" required achieving a certain level of physical recovery before security and social needs could be prioritized. I declined their offer to trade their pre-paid tickets to Park City for ones to see me since even at sea level the tests indicated that I was not capable of spending much time with them . It turned out that they needed this time together and shared it with me through stories and a photo magnet that smiled at me every time I opened our refrigerator.

Was my making my own tentative schedule a mistake? Heck no! As long as I understood it was "tentative" then thinking of it as "the spring of hope" (*The Tale of Two Cities*), helped my feeling that I was "Managing Your (MY) Rehabilitation Program WELL."

Lessons learned:

1. Goals must be flexible and subject to change and being able to breathe takes precedence over all other goals.

2. Altitude has a significant effect on our ability to breathe, which is why sleeping is common on airplanes where the pressure is the same as it is at 10,000 feet.

3. Evaluating doctors on their skills, not on their appearance, is important as is open and honest communications.

4. Focus on what a doctor tells you to do and not what they do in their personal lives.

CHAPTER 17. A BREATH OF FRESH AIR

My enthusiasm draining out of the same tube in my back as the fluid from my chest put this March in danger of following the saying that March was a change month that either entered like a lion and exited like a lamb, or vice versa. This March had entered like an aggressive lion and was slowly transitioning to the meek lamb just hoping to survive physically.

No question this was discouraging! On the day I reviewed all the alternatives, or as I came to call it, "I looked at the man in the mirror" (thanks Michael Jackson for the phrase), I did my best to change the subject for the rest of the day. It always amazed me how much differently everything looked the next day. On the day after canceling my Park City trip, I revisited my goals. My overriding goal remained to recover my independent lifestyle, but my maladies indicated that I needed to create new interim goals What were they?

My previous attempts to create a tentative schedule for recovery was just that: tentative, in that it was subject to unexpected events. But it definitely served its purpose. Of course it was a disappointment when problems interrupted its execution, but I used the word "tentative" to provide incentives while also reducing the disappointment if issues arose. The problem was not the goals: it was the execution.

Despite past disappointments, I again set my own interim goals of physically improving my breathing and emotionally readjusting my outlook. The pulmonologist had shown that my life was limited, unless and until, my breathing improved. I took the prescription drug and tried harder in formal rehab. On the treadmill I kept walking through the feelings that previously had stopped me; on the stationary bike I peddled harder; on the crank I refused to "cheat" by using my "other" arm as a leverage the way that some people do in arm wrestling. I increased the length and pace of my walks and only rested once while mounting the front steps of our building. I was sure I was making progress.

When the rehab nurse again said, "You are not making sufficient progress," I instantly felt my shoulders tighten. She continued, "It is time for more x-rays." This time I felt that I would fail: and I did.

This time I walked a little slower for my appointment with my pulmonologist. Into the hospital and down the all too familiar hallways to the same room where my now favorite pulmonologist was waiting. I knew the drill: strip to the waist, sit on the exam table, lean forward with my elbows on the still sliding silver tray and quietly pray while trying not to have my face show any emotions that might frighten Carol. At the doctor's direction, the nurse's felt tip pen started drawing a circle on my back. I was holding it together, barely, until the he said to the nurse, "You must be from pediatrics. Here we draw a much larger circle."

Doctors should remember that patients can hear their words and will provide their own interpretations. As the doctor drew a much larger circle, sweat burst out all over and I felt light-headed. I tried all my tricks. I asked myself what was the worst that could happen? Not good! I visualized my falling forward onto the tray on wheels that would roll away leaving me to fall on the floor with a tube sticking out of my back that would cause the glass jars to smash on top of me covering me with broken glass and the reddish brown stuff taken from my chest. The doctor asked, "Are you all right?"

"I don't know. Here feel my hand," I said twisting enough so that he could feel my right hand.

"It is very wet. What do you do when you are like this?"

"I don't know. This is the first time I have not been able to control my emotions."

When I later related this to my daughter, she said, "It's about time. Most of us were a lot younger than you are when we first learned this lesson. Why do you think I had a fear of flying?" In my case, the doctor said, "We had better reschedule when I can give you something to relax you first."

"Give me one now and begin as soon as it kicks in," I replied thinking that once I was emotionally prepared I did not want to delay. For example, when a dermatologist said he would schedule me to have a cancerous growth removed from my back in two weeks; I said "No, the stress of waiting will be too great. I am not getting off of this examination table until you cut it out." To his credit, when the doctor realized I was serious, he performed the surgery so I never had the time to feed my fears.

This time this doctor said, "We are not permitted to give you a controlled substance. I will give you a prescription for one."

"Am I supposed to sit here and wait while Carol goes to a pharmacy to have it filled?"

"Oh no, we will have to reschedule the procedure."

What? Was I really in a hospital with a physician who could perform surgical procedures and write prescriptions for a controlled substance but who could not administer the same controlled substance? Did the makers of the rules think it would be safer for me to take it at home rather than in the hospital? Did the rule makers not trust the security in hospitals who have security guards, but did trust security for drug stores without guards? Were the procedures for this "controlled" substance meant to control the substance, me or the doctor?

Ironically, my next appointment was on my birthday, March 28th,. But my rescheduling was out of the question after my heart stopping in the rescheduled stress test. So I began my birthday with a lawyers' maneuver of complying while also "hedging my bet" by keeping control by only taking one of the two pills prescribed for my nerves and, just in case, putting the other one in my pocket. Again, I stripped to the waist, sat on the sliding exam table, leaned forward placing my elbows on the sliding tray and looked at Carol. With the help of the pill I was holding it together. Then Carol said, "I feel faint. I need to wait in the waiting room" and left. Whoa, I knew she had, on occasion, fainted. Who would catch her if she collapsed in the hallway? Would anyone tell me? Would one pill now be sufficient?

I dared not take the other pill just in case I had to be able to help her. Searching for a distraction, I asked the doctor if my talking would not distract him, and after he said "no," I searched for a topic that I knew enough about to last the entire procedure. The only one that I knew that well was a prolonged discussion of my educational career. When he started cutting, I started babbling about my college career in a way that would do a woman in labor proud. I provided details that even I had never before focused on, starting with my studying engineering, then math, management, and when I got to my first year of law school, he said, "Time to change jars."

Oh no; he is only half-way through the two jar limit and I am almost through my college years. I had better go into even more excruciating detail, which I did so well that when the doctor emphatically again said "stop," I wondered if he meant my story or the test. Then he added, "We have reached the two liter limit." I briefly considered asking him if he would stand still while I finished my story. However, after he removed the tube, I followed a rule learned during my first argument before a judge: when a decision goes in your favor, shut up and leave. Being careful not to glance at the bottles, I put on my shirt with the pill still in the pocket, and intrepidly peered into the waiting room at Carol, who smiled over her magazine.

To prevent another fluid buildup, the pulmonologist prescribed prednisone from the class of corticosteroids that prevents the release of substances in the body that cause inflammation, which was why it was used to treat certain allergic and breathing disorders. All drugs have side effects, and the ones for prednisone included weakening immune systems used to fight infection. Another side effect was that it helped my courage, or the "quality or spirit that enables a person to face difficulty" (Macmillan Dictionary), as I hopefully watched March exit "like a lamb."

Lessons learned:

1. The path toward achieving an objective may be tentative and subject to setbacks that cannot distract from the ultimate goal.

2. Each person must understand their own emotional reactions and search for ways to control them. The responsibility is yours.

3. Once a course of medical treatment is selected, do everything you can to make it successful. If it fails, the doctor doesn't fail, you do.

CHAPTER 18. APRIL: A BREATH TAKING HOBSON'S CHOICE

As April arrived my breathing problems so dominated my thoughts that April first passed without any thoughts of the April Fool's day pranks or the light heartedness that typically accompanied this day in my youth in New Jersey. This April my breathing problems eliminated the conscious inclusion of any other topics. However, while the unconscious ones could be irrational, foolish, preposterous, or even ridiculous, they were real and could occur at strange times. This April mine were vivid romantic dreams. The cause of these dreams occurring at this time would remain a mystery. Logically it could have been the renewed blood flow through my repaired right carotid artery stimulating my feelings oriented right side of my brain, or a prednisone induced euphoria, or the moon's cycle, or the progression of the zodiac signs through Aries towards Taurus, or some other reasons. I, of course, knew as men universally always know: It was the rise of my masculinity that helped the emotional right side overwhelmed the logical left side.

In all the many hours we had spent together, the doctors, nurses and counselors, had discussed almost every aspect of my life, such as my health, breathing, financial, family, diet, exercise, and even bowel movements, in excruciating detail. The only forbidden topic seemed to be romantic intimacy. Throughout my life it had always been that way. I guess my mother thought it was up to my father, who apparently thought the one sentence of "Son, be careful as the men in our family are potent" said it all. But I don't think I was unique: it was a sign of the times. The advice Anne's parents gave her was, "We trust you to do the right thing," without a hint of what that was. Perhaps all the medical personnel had the same type of childhoods. Now it was I who wanted to "do the right thing:" I just didn't know what it was. Like a curious teenager, I started sneaking peaks at Carol. The sound of her shower began to bring visuals of the water streaming off her. My feelings when I hugged her in bed had progressed from helping me relax to keeping me awake. The axons carrying the voices back and forth in my brain went into overdrive starting with the message from the right side, "Hey fellow, I am getting some stimulus from down below," to which the left side responded, "The prednisone increases both enthusiasm and, ironically, impotency."

The dialogue continued with the right side saying, "Words can only be used to describe, not replace, feelings," and left side responded "I know prednisone creates false euphoria. I also know the male role requires an increase in blood pressure. Are you forgetting the pills you take each morning to prevent increases in your blood pressure?"

"Our same physician who prescribed the blood pressure pills also, without our asking, prescribed Viagra" was met with, "Yes, he did but the internet site Web.MD recommends regular heart patients first passing the stress test before taking Viagra. Besides, none of the literature helps since we are the rare exception with so extreme a post surgical breathing problem."

The debate continued with a preview of the future with the question, "Will you believe a website or a doctor who has actually examined us? When will you know?" followed by "I'll know when the euphoric effects of the prednisone wear off."

Right side, "Pills, hills, chills, thrills; at this point everything sounds sexy! Why do you always say 'no'?" was met by the left with, "Do you really want to bet on not causing a stroke or worse?"

The emotional side said "Every action is a bet of sorts. Monitor us and stop if it appears that we are threatening our life," was countered by, "What happens if we try and fail?"

Then in a tricky move, the arguments shifted to appeal to the emotional side of Carol by saying she has been a nurse for months and nurses have needs. Rather than worrying about the risks of trying and failing, worry about the risks of not showing you care enough to try.

It is difficult to say how many times a dialogue of this nature occurred before I said to Carol something like, "Honey, I miss the intimacy. I am not certain if it is medically safe, or even if it is possible while taking the blood pressure pills. If you are willing to risk failure, I am too."At least this is the theoretical discussion I had. In the heat of the moment I might have omitted all but the key points of "I want you but I am not certain of my capabilities." Carol's expression and prompt movements indicated that my actions were behind schedule. My analytical side tried to monitor my heart but soon lost the battle. Sometimes our bodies are capable of more than we give them credit for.

The physical and social aspects of intimate contact gave my self-image a lift, which was evident in the progress in my thoughts and feelings. After months of primarily thinking about myself, I had started thinking more about others and their lives. My life line to the world was the telephone, where my conversations were transitioning from just talking about me to wanting to talk more about other people and things. My world was expanding. At times I felt like a child learning to walk; at times, like a teenager, thinking about sports, girls and my future; at times, like an adult thinking about my future and, yes, sports and girls.

The prednisone slowly leaving my body took with it my feelings of euphoria. The lectures in the rehabilitation program were on a rotating eight week basis, and I assumed the exercise part of the formal rehab program was on the same eight week schedule which, for me, had elapsed weeks ago. Then, on April 10th, the three month anniversary of the beginning of my "One Heart-Two Lives" (capitalized as the name of this book), my hopes met reality when my rehab nurse sent me for another chest x-ray. I had no doubt that I would flunk: and I did.

When Carol and I entered our now favorite pulmonologist's office, we knew something was different. Gone were his hand shake and warm smile that had always extended through his full beard. His look through now dull eyes said it all: this meeting was different. His shoulders sagged. He looked as if he had aged ten years since out last time together. I worried that he was not well. Then he said, "Your chest x- rays showed the fluid has returned. I'm very sorry but there is nothing else that I can do for you."

What: had I heard him right? Needing a pulmonologist was scary: stumping one who also had a Ph.D. was frightening. The caring of this unmarried, childless doctor, who had tried so hard to enable me to see my children, was evident by the sagging in his shoulders and voice when he said, "There are two options. The first is to do nothing and lead a reduced lifestyle. You will never get any better and you could get much worse so quickly that it might be fatal. The second option is you can see a cardiac surgeon about having endoscopic surgery, which hopefully, would enable you to lead a normal life."

Some concepts arise so often that they are named after some classic example: a Hobson's choice is one of them. A Hobson's choice was when you were offered what appeared to be a choice but only one of the choices was feasible. It was named after Thomas Hobson (1544-1639), who owned a stable in Cambridge, England, where every customer wanted to rent only his best horses. Hobson wanted to distribute the rentals among all his horses equally, so he rotated the horses among the stalls and offered customers the choice of taking the horse in the stall nearest the door or none at all. For someone who really needed a horse it became a Hobson's Choice. One might wonder whether my unconscious desire for intimacy was a Hobson's Choice, but there was no doubt about lung surgery. My Hobson's Choice was to avoid surgery and live a dependent life in constant fear of my shortness of breath becoming even shorter and, perhaps, stopping; or having one of the last things I wanted, another surgery. How many surgeries could I survive? Now I understood the reason for the doctor's demeanor. He really cared. I asked, "Will the surgery work, and what are the risks?"

"The only surgeon in town who does this type of surgery is an expert," he responded. "You should ask him these questions at your appointment Friday." Carol and I sadly bid the caring doctor adieu.

Two days later, on Friday, the mystery surgeon entered my world. Or rather, I entered his. Based on his having practiced for years in Minnesota before moving to this town, I expected a semi-retired demeanor. This was not even close. His appearance and attitude were of a man in mid-career. Over the last several months I had become an incredible skeptic. For months a series of sincere, competent physicians had represented that they would solve my problems, but in reality, they didn't! I entered this surgeon's office determined to learn, before surgery, whether he really could solve my problems. I did not want to risk another surgery if my problems were insolvable. I started interviewing him like I would a witness for a trial. Not a friendly witness: a hostile one. I challenged everything he said by asking leading questions that were meant to annoy the surgeon, like it did witnesses, so he would blurt out an admission against his own interest. My manager had said I was the best he ever seen at this technique. I began by asking, "If my heart surgery was a success, why am I in your office today?"

The surgeon looked me in the eye and without hesitation, both good signs, said, "Your surgery was a success as it eliminated the blockage to your heart. You are here today because about 25% of the time during open heart surgery the lubricant on the sides of the lungs is lost. The vast majority of the time the patient's body naturally reproduces it. In less than 1/2 of 1%, or in less than 1 heart patient in every 200, the body does not reproduce the lubricant. You are one of these."

I liked the idea of a straight answer and under my fear I knew the surgery had given my one heart an opportunity to serve two lives. But I was overwhelmed at again defying the odds. This time it was ½ of 1% of 25% of the 3% survival rate for heart stoppage preceded by the 1 in 100,000 who have a serious negative event during a stress echo test. Quickly the odds of anyone having my set of experiences was reaching 1 in 100 million. How many times can I defy the odds?

I asked, "How does your procedure work, and will the fluid return as it has several times after my chest was drained?"

"I will do an endoscopic surgical procedure where I will enter your chest and glue your lungs into a position where they can open and close without friction. It cannot return, as there will not be any room."

Instead of asking the success rate, I asked the opposite, "How many times has the procedure failed?" The surgeon seemed to reflect before replying, "I cannot remember a single time when it did not work."

This was encouraging but hostile witnesses sometimes had short memories, so I asked, "How many of these do you do in a year? "I really don't know," he said with a smile, and perhaps even a laugh, before turning to Carol and asking, "Is he always like this?" Carol smiled back and said, "No, sometimes he is much worse. He is an attorney!"

While everybody laughed, including me, the math major part of me was doing a quick calculation. If my situation arose once in every 200 heart surgeries, and he performed 250 heart surgeries a year, than my situation arises a little more than once a year. This was not confidence building! But my Hobson's Choice was whether or not to trust this surgeon who did not seem to have all the experience I preferred and either not have the surgery or travel hundreds of miles in search of a surgeon with that experience. How desperate was I to quickly have the surgery?

So I said, "Can I wait and if a problem arises, then have the surgery?"

"No, you are near the end of a tight window for being eligible for this type of surgery. Once the window closes any problems will require another open chest surgery."

I asked, "What is the soonest you can schedule me?"

He replied, "Does next Wednesday, April 25th, or Thursday work for you?"

Following my practice of selecting the first date so, in the event of a problem, there was another date available, I said, "Please schedule me for Wednesday; and thank you for handling my questions so well." My thinking like a lawyer meant that I systematically evaluated the alternatives, but once I made a decision to become supportive of my new teammate. Besides, I would have to be crazy to risk alienating a surgeon who the next time I saw him would have a scalpel in his hand.

Over the weekend as I mentally prepare for my latest surgery, the disappointment in the face and words of the pulmonologist when he said, "I can't help you," haunted me.

On the day before my surgery, as soon as I walked into rehab the facial expression of the normally upbeat nurse L. told me something was horribly wrong. She said, "Yesterday your pulmonologist was found dead in his bed. Apparently he died in his sleep. He was 53."

This hit me hard. I really liked this caring, competent and compassionate man. I had no idea that just a few days ago when we said adieu that would it would be our final adieu. His being ten years younger than me was a dose of reality that reminded me of the time I read that the projected life expectantly for trial lawyers was 56. "He died of the same condition he was treating me for," I blurted out as I suddenly felt very mortal. What chance did I have if the expert in the subject in which I needed help, breathing, had died of breathing problems? The best that I came up with was that I was still standing and would continue to manage my own rehabilitation program. So to the memory of my pulmonologist friend, I said, "Thanks for keeping me alive. I am sorry you did not follow your own advice, but I will: thank you for caring and adieu." Little did I know that later I would have to repeat this process when my expert on my other main issue, managing stress, fell victim to stress at approximately the same age as the good doctor.

Sometimes what at first appears to be a difficult decision transforms, once the facts are understood, into a Hobson's Choice, with only one acceptable alternative, and are there any stronger drives than for breathing or for intimacy? My heart surgery offered me a second chance to live and now my lung surgery offered a "second" chance for "Managing Your (my) Rehabilitation Program WELL" to help make my "One Heart-Two Lives" a reality: Bring it on!

Lessons Learned:

1. Satisfying our physiological needs takes priority over all other needs. When the need for air fails to meet a minimum standard, obtaining it becomes more important than all other needs.

2. Understanding our feelings and making them work for us can be powerful in keeping our objectives in mind.

3. Organize your questions before meeting a physician and ask the tough questions, as long as you ask them politely.

4. Recognize when you have a Hobson's choice.

5. Evaluate physicians on their expertise and competence, rather than their "bedside manner." Once you decide on a physician, consider him or her your teammate and do whatever you possibly can to assist in making their efforts successful.

6. Be proactive: It helps you remain positive and avoid feeling like a victim. Staying positive may, or may not, help our subconscious keep us alive but it gives you hope. Comply with your doctor's orders.

CHAPTER 19. LUNG SURGERY WITH A TWIST

I awoke, startled! I kept trying to run but my feet were so heavy that I could barely walk. Dreams are basically stories and images our mind creates while we sleep, and can make you feel happy, sad or scared while being confusing or rational (webMD). Was mine related to today's surgery?

The ups and downs of my roller coaster life were now coming at break neck speed. One day I was thinking of romance; the next one I was interrogating a surgeon as a hostile witness; then mourning the death of a new friend and now, once again, I am a humble future patient hoping to survive another surgery. I did feel that the end was near since if this surgery failed then so did my chances of "Managing Your (my) Rehabilitation Program WELL," since this was my final option within the traditional medical community.

I told myself "just one more time—the finish line is in sight. You have come a long way and all that is left is correcting your body's rushing too much fluid to compensate for the friction caused by the lack of lubricant on your lungs." This surgery could be the end of my suffocating myself. My trusted pulmonologist, in what turned out to be his last days, admitted defeat and referred me to the only surgeon within a hundred miles who could perform my needed Thoracoscopy Pleurod surgery. My aggressive "examination" of this surgeon had quickly shifted to friendly when I realized that I trusted him to be able to prevent my again becoming a walking time bomb. My Hobson's Choice disintegrated into one of timing. If I delayed even a week or so, and the fluid buildup continued as it already had done twice, and I survived, the only remedy would then be another open chest surgery.

Thoracoscopy surgery: This surgery involved cutting three narrow openings in my chest. One for inserting an endoscope, which was a narrow tube with a mirror or camera attached, another for the surgical instrument to diagnose and perform therapeutic services on the lungs, the area between the lungs (mediastinum) or the area surrounding the lungs (pleura), and the third for inserting tubing that would be left open so the fluid and air could drain after surgery (healthcommunities.com). It would be much less intrusive than open chest surgery, but it still was a surgery that required a general anesthetic. The projected hospital stay was 2-5 days (mayoclininc.com).

A welcomed development in recent years was the elimination of the requirement for the patient to be admitted to the hospital the night before surgery simply to ensure that the patient did not eat. Not eating was an easy choice once my research identified the reason for the no eat rule was to prevent the anesthetic from causing vomiting or food particles lodging in lungs, which might result in serious complications up to, and including, death. The remaining question of whether fasting included not taking my prescription blood pressure pills had been answered by a physician instructing me to take them with water, which I did, but without taking any of my normal vitamins. Per instructions, Carol and I arrived at 9:00 A.M. and were taken to a regular patient's room to wait for the 1:45 scheduled surgery. Time soon drained as quickly out of the figurative hour glass as glue would on a cold day.

By 1 P.M., every foot step in the hall drew my expectant eyes to the door. At 2 P.M., I took some solace from thinking that the delays in my scheduled time were because the operating room was needed for patients with more serious problems. At 3 P.M., I started my countdown: bathroom visit, pace the room, take off street clothes, bathroom visit (nerves are powerful), put on hospital gown, bathroom visit, pace the room, bathroom visit with Carol's voice coming through the door, "they are here." It was funny how their arrival cured my impatience. Now I moved very slowly onto a gurney so an orderly could wheel me out the door and down the hall with clean ceilings. When we reached the door the pre-opt room, instead of saying "good bye," which might be a bad omen, I said to Carol, "I'll see you later." My gurney ride entered this pre-op room where the nurse, without asking about any out-of-body experiences, pushed me through the now familiar swinging doors. On the table, I took a deep breath to relax and after 91 there was nothingness.

Post surgery: When I opened my eyes, my first thought, as always, was I am alive. I was in a bed with a wall on my right side and an empty bed on my left. With every deep breath the pain in my right side, halfway up my rib cage, far exceeded my threshold for pain, which was a lawyer's way of saying "it hurt like H--l." I remembered the story of the fellow who said to his doctor, "When I raise my arm like this it hurts," to which the doctor in the story replied, "Then don't raise your arm like that," I resolved to not take any deep breaths although I did wonder about the irony of not taking deep breaths after a surgery to enable me to take deep breaths. There was a clear plastic, flexible tube sticking in my right side halfway up my rib cage at exactly the spot that hurt so much. What a coincidence! A nurse entered and after telling me it was a drainage tube that led to a glass bottle on the floor where the "stuff" would be collected, she continue, "Keep the drainage tube from pulling out. If it pulls out it might cause a 'pneumothorax,' which is where one or both of your lungs collapses." Now there was an incentive to sit still since the tube just reached the floor.

There were two bandages on my right side just below my rib cage. A really good sign was that there was "only" one other tube; an intravenous tube, or "IV," in my left wrist. My plan to sit very still because of the pain only lasted until a nurse entered and handed me the Voldyne while instructing me to repeatedly blow as hard as I could in order to manually re-open my lungs as quickly as possible. I was not only weak, which was typical as the recovery specifies only "light lifting" for weeks afterwards, but also drained and helpless.

A little later a nurse pulled the pale green curtain that extended from the ceiling to about two feet above the floor, down the track in the ceiling that separated my bed from the other bed in the room, while saying, "You are getting a roommate." A few minutes later all the other patients on my floor heard my new roommate make his entrance with a yell of "What kind of a hotel is this?" My glance of him as he passed the end of the curtain indicated that he appeared to be in his 60's, thin approximately four inches shorter than my six feet, with short gray hair, and surprisingly, was still dressed in street clothes.

He proceeded to yell at the nurse standing a foot from him, "You lousy bitch. Where is my girl friend?" The nurse politely said, "Sir, I don't know where your girl friend is," to which he responded, "What kind of a jail is this?" These accusations, which always included some words not fit to write here, became his routine. Somehow, to the nurses' credit, they remained calm. But I did not. From where I came from, if you talked like that to anyone, you had better be prepared to "back it up."

His next salvo was, "I'll give you ten minutes to produce my girl friend or I'll beat the f—k out of you." Besides being obnoxious, his use of the word "produce" sounded familiar, although I did not immediately place it. When the nurse re-entered the room, he yelled, "Let me out of this jail, you bitch, or I will seek a writ of habeas corpus."

Oh no, now I remembered why the word "produce" sounded familiar. It was for the same reason "writ of habeas corpus" did. They were terms with particular meaning in the legal profession. In litigation, requests for opponents to provide documents or other things were phrased in terms of having them "produce" them. Writs of habeas corpus, which in Latin means "you have the body," are used to require a person under arrest to be brought before a judge to guarantee the person had an opportunity to defend themselves in court. The Supreme Court later expanded this right to include having counsel (Miranda v Arizona, 384 U.S. 436 (1966).

Just my luck: my new roommate was a lawyer. While many of my friends are lawyers, none were not this type of lawyer. I have no idea what this guy had been like before his obvious dementia, but now I was trapped in a hospital room with a disoriented, obscene, distasteful, offensive, nasty, threatening lawyer with a strong voice that he demonstrated every few minutes: for hours. Sometimes, he demanded to be released from a hotel; and sometimes from jail; but never from a hospital. Every time I started to feel sorry for his dementia, he would yell at a nurse some threat containing the "f" word. Finally, a nurse said, "Sir, you are in a hospital and you are disturbing the patient in the next bed."

"There is no patient in the next bed. But if there was one, then I would beat him for complaining," was his next yell. That got my attention. I dared not follow the prescribed post surgical directions to sleep, or even make any noise while using the Voldyne. I felt vulnerable and defenseless. From my quick glance of him, I concluded that during normal times I could take him. But after my surgery, even if I held him off, the tubes sticking out my sides would injure me and might collapse a lung. Minimally, a fight would surely violate the reasons for the "light lifting" instructions. I looked for a weapon. The only thing even remotely useful thing that I could reach was the glass jar on the floor where the tube from my chest was draining reddish brown fluid. I tried, unsuccessfully to reach it. Maybe in a crisis I could stretch. I had better not dose off.

Over the next several hours every patient on the hospital floor were constantly victims of his vocal rages. Obviously he did not have my type of breath limiting surgery. Around midnight he got out of bed, and as I cocked my right arm, he walked to the end of the curtain and, without looking in my direction, walked out the door while announcing, "I am leaving this hotel." What a relief to hear him walk across the hallway and get on an elevator. I, of course, said nothing. Perhaps because of the sudden quiet, a nurse sounded an alarm.

Unfortunately, a short time later, a uniform security guard brought him back and forced him onto the bed. His threats of violence became so vivid that I thought he would attack the soft looking guard who stayed at the foot of his bed. The guard repeatedly said to him, "Sir, you are disturbing your roommate." The repeated response was, "I don't have a roommate. But if I did, I would beat him for complaining." I didn't say I was an attorney because his attitude almost guaranteed that his relationships with other attorneys were really bad.

When the security guard left, I called the nurse and told her blood was again running out the side of the I.V. in my left arm and I feared for my safety. For the second time the nurse added tape around the I.V. and removed the tube from my chest and took the glass jar with her when she left. "Great," I thought, "My I.V. is leaking and there goes my only possible weapon."

The yelling continued as the nurse returned and held my hand. In just a few minutes, her call for assistance led to the arrival of a male dressed in hospital scrubs. His appearing to be in good shape was soon tested as his attempts to reason with the guy ended with his winning a wrestling match. He managed to fasten my roommate to some sort of portable frame and then left. My roommate twisted so much that I could see his feet hanging off the bed but the frame apparently kept him from completely getting off the bed: at least for now.

The yelling continued. Around 3 A.M., the nurse returned and said, "Stand up, grab your I.V. stand and follow me." Having not slept in the almost 12 hours since my surgery, my movements were unstable as I rolled out of bed and took small, wobbly, painful steps past the danger zone behind the now fast moving nurse. Worried that eye contact might trigger an outburst; I never looked at my roommate while flashing him, and every other person we passed on our way to another room. After I collapsed onto the bed by the door, I wondered why we had not done this sooner since, obviously, there was a bed available.

The sun pouring in the window woke me. When I finally could focus on blowing into the Voldyne, the pain was so great that I asked a nurse, "Why after surgery to open my lungs, do I have to do it manually?"

"Because you will stay in the hospital until you do," she persuasively said. I later learned that the longer answer was that the surgery made it "possible" for my lungs to open all the way, but only after I first "forced" them open with deep breaths and the sooner a patient starts this, the easier and less painful it is. Almost 18 hours after surgery I was finding it neither easy nor painless.

Two white-coats entered. My endoscopic surgeon said he was pleased that my surgery was successful and my role was to continue to blow into the Voldyne and rest, neither of which had been possible until now. He was accompanied by my carotid surgeon, with whom during my numerous visits I had exchanged stories of our times at Temple University, his in residency and mine teaching management. This time he smilingly said, "I understand that you shared a room last night with one of my patients." My saying, "Congratulations if you were treating him for shortness of breath," made him laugh.

At lunch time, Carol and a nurse observed the tears running down my cheeks as I blew into the Voldyne. Immediately the nurse said, "That shot we gave you for pain is not working" before leaving and returning with pills. The pain instantly became manageable. I guess the confusion of last night had distracted the nurses from paying attention to my recovery; which, in effect, was just now starting almost 24 hours after my surgery. As the story of last night made the rounds and the head nurse stopped in to apologize, which I really appreciated, I said, "I am surprised that this happened here since your hospital was so highly recommended." She said, "By whom?"

"By a board member of this hospital," I said giving his name. The nurse asked, "Do you know him?" My wife, who was sitting there, said "Yes, I work closely with him and he will be surprised at my husband's story."

The nurse left and quickly returned saying, "We have an opening in my favorite room. It even has a view of a tree. Let me move you there." The room was, indeed, a nice way to obtain the rest prescribed for post surgical patients. The next morning after I achieved my first triumph over the Voldyne, and starting my second day of the 2-5 days recommended by the Mayo Clinic, I was discharged.

As I was wheeled out of the hospital, I thought back to that faithful day at Clemson University when Dr. Clinton Whitehurst challenged me with the words, "Few people in life are given a second chance, and even fewer take advantage of it. I hope you are one." Thank you, Dr. Whitehurst, for these words that even after forty years will again help to inspire me to keep "Managing Your (my) Rehabilitation Program WELL." After all, there is no more important second chance than to make "One Heart---Two Lives" successful. That certainly was, and would be, my plan.

Lessons Learned:

1. Breathing is so important that taking calculated risks to improve it may be worthwhile.

2. Any threat to your physical security is serious.

3. Sleep is necessary for our bodies to recover from surgery.

4. Attitude can make a difference in every aspect of life. Whether our days are good or bad usually does not depend on "what" we do as much as "how" we do them.

5. The doctors and nurses will do what they can for our physical recovery but the mental and emotional sides are up each of us.

6. When making a choice, evaluate and understand the alternatives before agreeing to any treatment; especially surgery.

CHAPTER 20. MAY: A TIME TO CELEBRATE?

May 1st? I had been so caught up in my condition and recent hospital adventures that seeing May 1 appear in my Day Timer caused me to lean back and reflect: Did the recent surgery mean it was time to call for more help, or to celebrate?

The very words "May Day" are derived from the French expression "*venez m'aider*," meaning "come to help me," which came to be internationally recognized as indicating a life threatening emergency; particularly when used as a radio message from mariners and aviators and, in some countries, by police forces and fire fighters.

On January 10th, my *venez m'aider* had been answered by physicians. Eleven days later I left the tender care in the hospital and entered the same type of care at home as the calendar for January closed. February's tentative plans to see my family in March continued despite setbacks. March's hopes survived the first setback before the second one drained them faster than the liquid through the tubes inserted in my back. April's prednisone high experienced a decline so steep that it exceeded the capabilities of a pulmonologist with a Ph.D. in chemistry. Should May begin with another *venez m'aider* or a celebration?

In 1958 President Eisenhower initiated the U.S. celebrating May 1st as "Law Day," and Congress "made it official" by declaring it "a special day of celebration by American people in appreciation of their liberties and rededication to the ideas of equality and justice under law." For these reasons, as well as The American Bar Association pronouncing that Law Day was a celebration of "the freedoms all Americans share." My career was built on preserving these freedoms for others. Now I was fighting to again personally enjoy the rights of "life, liberty and the pursuit of happiness" (Declaration of Independence).

Some say the custom of celebrating May 1st began with the festival of Flora," the Roman goddess of flowers, while others connect it to pagan customs in the Germanic and Gaelic countries.

As the years transitioned from B.C. to A.D., the festivities in the Northern Hemisphere transitioned to ones celebrating a spring festival. While the reasons people celebrated this day varied over the centuries, what remained constant was that much like the hundreds of years passing between celebrations surrounding the rock structure known as Stonehenge; the tradition to celebrated continued. I understood that it may have been the vibrations I felt in that rock structure near Salisbury, England, but my understanding of why May 1st was limited to one of appreciating that while the reasons changed, the celebrations persevered.

Indeed, in 1894, the Marxists started celebrating May 1st, as the International Workers Holiday, with the words indicated by the lines, "With a message of hope and strife, Raise the Maypole aloft with its garlands...Together pull, strong and united" (The Workers Maypole).

On this May Day, my question was whether I had progressed to where I could shift my reasons for celebrating this day from representing a call for assistance to reclaiming the ability to celebrate it for the reason initiated in the U.S. by President Eisenhower?

I hoped to although all the ups and downs of the past months had diminished my willingness to celebrate. After I returned to rehab, I again became cautiously optimistic until, once again, I was rocked by the nurse's eight short words: "It is time for your stress echo test." She continued, "The final step in your rehabilitation program is for you to re-take and pass the test that you were finishing when your heart stopped."

The emotional right side of my brain screamed, "What? Are you seriously asking me to re-take the same test that ended my first life?"

The analytical left side responded, "Relax. We just celebrated on May Day our personal freedoms for such things as being able to refuse to take the test and just walk away."

Right side, "Either way I am frightened to leave our tiny, familiar world that has shrunk to just the rehab center and our condo. I take this is not weird as many patients in therapy become dependent on their therapist and even some harden prisoners on friendly guards as evidence by the Stockholm Syndrome."

Left side, "We are going to be free of the program, but what is our greatest internal fear?"

This technique of thinking of extremes and, if I could handle these, then understanding that I could handle anything less usually helped my decision making. I remembered the fear I felt when reading a book written by G. Gordon Liddy. When he was a teenager, to overcome his fear of rats, he caught one, cooked it over a camp fire, and ate it (*Autobiography of G. Gordon Liddy*). He later demonstrated his lack of fear when, as a security advisor to President Nixon, he carried out a chore that led to prison time. This was such a strong sign of facing a fear in order to overcome it, that I adopted "let's eat a rat" as my silent rallying cry when I faced tough situations. Why silent? Because I understood Carol's never warming up to this cry. Her childhood memories included one of her three brothers sneaking up behind her and placing a mouse he had caught on their farm on her shoulder. So I silently asked, "Should I eat the rat or face a lifetime of fearing the uncertainty?

When phrased a certain way, sometimes questions answered themselves. However, this time getting ready was different: I was not oblivious to the risks, there were no attempted jokes about Carol taking out insurance on me for just that day, and I did not dress for a subsequent workout at the YMCA. This time was similar in that I declined Carol's offer to accompany me; but not for the reason of not needing support. This time I replied, "Thanks, but something I have to do by myself." This time my old Jag started right up, as it had every time since that December day of my scheduled test.

The staff in the Cardiology Department indicated that I should take a seat and join the others in the waiting room. I took a seat but did not join the others as I now felt the same way as I had felt on a surgical gurney: I was a group of one!

This was my walk down the hall. This was my test. I did not bother to read the release form as I now knew that the odds of 100,000 to one against having a heart attack during the test were not much consolation for the one.

Just the sight of the trend mill caused my head and hands to burst into cold sweats. Acting bravely can be vastly different from feeling brave. As this team of technicians, who I did not recognize (thank goodness) was wiring me up, I smiled at the brief, surprise visit by a face from my reduced world of rehab, nurse L.: thanks again. Wired up, and the treadmill started moving faster and the angle increased, I realized that I would never again relinquish responsibility for any test. I would determine how long and hard I would try. Then it was over.

During the recovery time, I decided that if I needed to take a breath, I would, even if it violated the instructions and invalidated the test. The words, "You passed," were music to my ears as I realized that I had neither felt tightness in my chest nor perspired profusely. The results confirmed physically what my taking the responsibility for, and during, the test had already confirmed: I was ready to take responsibility for my life. Had my silent call of "May Day" been answered by my emotions?

I remembered some other times when my emotions instantly stimulated a greater physical performance. When I worked in Delaware, my lunch time breaks were great examples. Just walking down those cement steps from Market Street to the Brandywine River Valley caused my feet to start jogging next to the canal. To me entering the river valley was like entering another eco system that, as the seasons changed, offered an opportunity to appreciate the beauty of the kaleidoscope of colors and shapes as the falling leaves exposed the unclad beauty of the trees and river.

To this history buff, this canal, which had been dug by the DuPont company to supply power for their dynamite and gun powder mills, served as a reminder of the contributions to our freedoms the Brandywine had witnessed; from the farmers fighting for our independence during the Revolutionary War's battle of the Brandywine Creek in 1777; to the DuPont's using its water to supplying the gun powder to fight every battle for freedom; to the dynamite used by the military, as well as miners, to protect and enrich our country. As my thoughts would flow back in time and up the river, I visualized the Wyatts, first N.C. and then Andrew, illustrating manuscripts, like *Treasure Island*, before shifting to the beauty of their surroundings along the Brandywine near Chadds Ford, Pennsylvania, where they removed everything else from their canvases in order to expose the unclad beauty of things like old barns, windows, rail fences and Andrew's neighbor Helga. My isolation in rehab had provided the luxury of the opportunity to further explore these thoughts.

Money Shows: While I was enjoying my new found introspection, Carol was burned out and needed a change. The flyer for the Money Show in Las Vegas offered an opportunity for such a change. We wondered if our attending, for the first time, this show would also help renew a much needed source of income. So on a warm day in May, we put the top down on Carol's convertible and started the 280 mile ride. As only easterners would do, we put the top down for our first ride through the dessert. I was unprepared for the difficulty I would have in breathing in the hot, dry air whisking by at 75 miles an hour. Passing the sign stating that we were at an altitude of 4,000 feet was a grim reminder of my failing the tests run by my late pulmonologist. If we tried, without stopping, to put the top up it would blow off, and there was no place to safely stop. Then the car in front of us, and all cars, stopped. I must have been the only person ever to be thrilled to be in a traffic jam in the middle of the dessert. Putting the top up improved my breathing.

Entering Las Vegas after months of a world of back and forth from home-to-rehab was jolting. The "in your face" glitz and glitter indoctrination was undoubtedly less than the one Rip Van Winkle experienced when waking after sleeping for twenty years (fictional story by Washington Irving (1783-1859)), but undoubtedly more than the first time one of the Wyatt's walked into the crowd at Buckley's Tavern.

While walking into our hotel/casino, I related to the comments said about the economist Thurston Veblen, who never fully participated in life, of, "He views the world as an outsider." Maybe this comparison was not so outlandish as the casinos can be seen from outer space. Internally they are designed so that to go anywhere, such as the Money Show, you had to walk through their gambling tables and machines. To hide my weakness, I faked an interest in the gambling tables but when we reached a stretch of bored dealers standing behind empty tables: my masquerade was over.

Money Shows provided many things---thousands of people simultaneously searching for ideas on investing from each other, speakers hawking their newsletters, computer programs, mutual funds, stocks, or any number of investment services or products, and exhibitors hoping to attract attention through the flash and flesh of their booths--- although a place to relax was not one of them. Attendees eyes and ears were constantly alert for that one tidbit of a conversation, either theirs or the persons around them, that would lead to riches. The prime target for tips were the people wearing suits or sport coats, which were only the speakers and one other person who was wearing a blue blazer because of his increased sensitivity to air conditioning. The intrigue my blazer created was enhanced by my lung issues making me one of the few attendees who was not constantly talking. When a couple joined us standing at a table said, "I see from your name tag you are from the upscale town of Santa Barbara. Any tips you can share?" His comments solidified that sometimes wisdom is attributed to one who does not feel compelled to brag, particularly if he is wearing a blazer at a Money Show. Not being able to pass up this opportunity to have some fun, I leaned in and whispered, "Take deep breaths and stay vertical. Now, if you will excuse us" and walked away to a chorus of "Do you mean pausing between trades, or digging deep within a particular industry or stock, or structured options or bonds…"

The various meanings of May Day illustrated the question of whether this month would involve a call for help or an exercise of freedoms? To face my fears and take the previously fatal test, I needed help. But by finding it within myself I was exercising, and enhancing, my freedom to live independently. I was realizing that a benefit of having the stimulus of my world reduced during rehabilitation was that it provided an opportunity for me to better understand, and appreciate, the internal, as well as the external, beauty of persons, places and things, that surrounded me. These were the essence of my life. The trick, then, for me, was that as my world expanded "To thine own self be true," (Hamlet, Shakespeare). Las Vegas was a test as it goes to extremes to distract visitors from staying true to themselves.

Lessons Learned:

1. The physical impact on attitude was obvious but the reverse, the impact of attitude on physical recovery, was also powerful.

2. Physical recovery can serve as a base for the mental and emotional sides of security, relationships and intellectual interests.

CHAPTER 21. JUNE: A TIME TO LAUGH, THINK AND CRY

June arrived full of hope. May not having "a step backwards" for every "two steps forward" indicated that the surgeon had not only withstood my cross examination, but also managed to deliver as promised, despite the attempts at disruption by my hospital roommate. Clearly, the time had come for me to exit the protections of my rehab world. But I wanted to do it slowly in order to secure the values that I had "discovered" while in my world of reduced distractions, which is a way of saying my "small world" without stimulating the song that is played 1,200 times a day in the ride at Disneyland.

So June found me with some trepidations, a gentle word for anxieties, apprehensions or just plain fear. Fear, not at leaving my small world or at re-entering my former larger one, but in how I did it. It was staying true to my values while expanding my world. I managed the challenges of responding by facing, rather than avoiding, the fear of my stress test. The Money Show in Las Vegas was confirmation that I was ready to re-enter the larger world.

My hopes of slowly expanding my world imploded in early June when Carol said, "Brent, would you like to attend the Mellon Bank Client Advisory Board (CAB) meeting in New York with me?"

So many thoughts fighting to be heard in my mind. New York, the largest, most exciting and most overwhelming city in our country. I learned to love New York while spending so many weeks in the World

Trade Center while winning the longest trial in the history of OSHA. I learned on the first day how stressful this trial would be when listening to OSHA's opening statement sent my back into such bad spasms that I could not stand for the lunch break. The nights, such as the first one when I called a doctor to my room, were a combination of a quick dinner followed by hours in what we labeled our "war room" where we prepared for the next day. As the trial continued, to ease the stress of the long, hotly contested trial days, I dragged myself up before sunrise and joined the amazingly large number of other joggers in Central Park. While this venue was vastly different from my lunch time runs on the Brandywine, these runs became the best part of the day and provided a pleasant distraction during even the most boring witnesses, which for a lawyer always means the other side's witnesses. On the non-trial days, we learned how great N.Y. is for walking to places such as Jackson and Times Squares.

As much as I liked N.Y., this time my thoughts were "No, I don't want to risk it," but since this was a big deal for her my words were, "Yes; if I get too tired, I can rest."

Flying: I reasoned that I had passed the stress test and survived the trip to Las Vegas, so I hoped I was ready for this challenge. For my first flight since "flunking" the oxygen utilization test and canceling my trip to Park City, I had planned a short one at a low altitude as a test, such as the flight from Santa Barbara to LAX, the Los Angeles airport, which was the first leg of our N.Y. trip. I thought I could survive any breathing problems on this flight and, if none, take the second leg to N.Y.

The agent at the ticket counter in Santa Barbara eliminated my contingency plan with the words, "Last night's fog prevented the incoming flight from arriving, so your plane is at LAX. The flight crew is on their way to LAX in a taxi and there is a bus waiting for you outside." I boarded the bus wondering: is this an omen?

We arrived at LAX, checked our bags and took our seats that were so close to the opaque wall separating the sections that I could not fully extend my legs. While the other passengers slowly boarded, the wall started to creep closer. My skin felt clammy. Breathing became difficult. I felt like there were bugs inside me. I tried distraction techniques but this time it raised thoughts of my pulmonologist ordering oxygen for my flight to Park City based on the thinner air at higher altitudes. I remembered him saying that the air pressure inside commercial airplanes is set to be equivalent to that of the pressure at 10,000 feet. Normally, people can handle this without extra oxygen: could I?

My test in March had indicated that at the altitude of 7,000 feet, my oxygen utilization rate would be only 58%. In the hospital when my rate dropped to "only" 91% they had given me oxygen. I felt my recent surgery must have improved my rate. But what if at a pressure of 7,000 or 10,000 feet my rate had improved but only to 70% or 80%? For the first time I questioned why hadn't I requested another test before flying, and I guessed that it was because the confusion of my pulmonologist dying. I hoped this would be a harmless oversight.

The flight attendant's standard announcement penetrated my thoughts with, "in the event of a decrease in the cabin pressure an oxygen mask will drop." I looked up at the closed compartment overhead. Would the mask drop if I was the only person who needed oxygen? If not, would I be able to pry it down in the minute or two before passing out? If yes, would any air flow or would the entire plane have to be in danger for the oxygen to flow?

As the wall crept closer, the attendant deviated from the usual script by adding, "Due to a back up at the airport in New York, in five minutes we are going to pull away from the gate and park on the tarmac for at least two hours." I felt he was talking directly to me. I knew the already shrinking air flow would be further reduced as we sat on the ground. If I could not handle it, did I have an exit plan for after the plane pulled away from the gate? Could I push the attendants out of the way and jump off the plane? How will I get the door open? Doors on planes are not close to the ground, so if I jump will I land on an asphalt runway in the middle of a busy airport with maybe a broken leg? Sweat ran down my face as I visualized trying to dodge huge planes.

I had no idea that many people fear being overwhelmed with such anxieties during a flight; particularly after a significant life changing event, like a birth, death, marriage, divorce or graduation (Anxiety and Depression Association of America). Heart surgery certainly qualified as one of these events. A phobia is defined as an altered state of consciousness; with symptoms including sweating, numbness in the hands and feet and a pounding heart, much like a heart attack (www.nytimes 07/24/2007).

All I knew was for the first time in my life I could not control my fear. How long ago was the attendant's warning that we had five minutes? I spoke my first words to Carol; "I'm getting off." Without waiting for her response, I rushed up the aisle ready to fight to keep that door open. I was getting off this plane. When I reached the front, I was relieved. The door was still open, and I was taller and boarder than the male attendant so there was no way he could keep me on this plane. Taking a deep breath, I said to him, "Thanks for the warning. I'm a heart patient." Hearing these words made me realize how scared I was since I never referred to myself as heart patient. Now I would say whatever it took to get off. The attendant responded, "That's why I made the announcement."

Carol arrived and breathlessly asked, "What are you doing?" My heart was speeding so fast that I knew no one would be able to understand me. Maneuvering myself between the attendant and the open door to make sure he could not stop me from getting off, I took a deep breath while saying, "I'm getting off this plane. I cannot sit on the runway for two hours."

"You can't get off. We have to get to New York for meetings," Carol said, having been given no warnings that my acting so out-of-character was not by choice.

"You have to get to New York for meetings. I don't. This was meant to be a fun trip for me, and it is not fun anymore," I said, to which she replied "I can't get off. I have a schedule to keep."

"You can do whatever you like. I'm getting off this plane— now," I replied standing a little taller so the attendant would realize he should not try to stop me. To his credit he stood quietly listening to Carol asking, "How will you get to New York?"

"I have no idea. Perhaps I will not go," I said with one eye on the door. Her next question was, "How will you get back to Santa Barbara?"

"I have no idea. I'll walk the hundred miles if I have to," I responded, realizing she had no idea how strong my anxieties were. She asked, "What about our luggage," to which the attendant interjected, "We cannot get your luggage off the plane." Wondering why she was talking about "stuff" at a time like this, I said, "We'll deal with it later. I don't care if we throw it away. There is nothing in my bag that I can't replace. I am getting off this plane," I said over my shoulder as I stepped off the plane. "I will discuss anything you like in the terminal."

Carol followed me saying, "Only one other couple got off." My response was, as it would be the other thirty times I would hear this comment, "I don't care what anyone else does. I made the right decision."

Once we were safely in the terminal, all my systems returned to normal, and I calmly said, "I agreed to fly on the basis that we would begin with a short test flight. I fought through my anxieties that it being canceled was a bad omen. On this plane, I was already having trouble getting air and feeling more confined by the minute. I lost control when the announcement was made that we would sit for hours on the tarmac where I know they reduce the already skimpy oxygen flow. I thought my considering jumping might frighten her, so instead I said, "I had to get off that plane at any cost. Luggage can be replaced."

Now that my panic attack had subsided, I decided that there was a risk that the longer my fear of flying festered; the harder it would be to ever fly again. Using the Marines' concept of "advancing in another direction," I decided to "eat the rat" in smaller bites. So I said, "let's go to the airline desk and see if there are shorter flights that will get us from L.A. to N.Y.

The ticket agent was suspicious of unusual request of more stops until my explanation about the announcement on the plane triggering my claustrophobia. I would never know why it emerged at this particular time, except that so far in my second life I was much more emotional. My request brought back memories and a new appreciation for the time I booked my daughter, Hollie, on a non-stop flight from San Diego to Philadelphia. She called saying she could not board it and requesting that I break it into smaller segments. Even before 9/11 the agent was suspicious of my request for at least two stops until I explained that it was to accommodate Hollie's fear of flying, which was exacerbated by her asthma. The agent not only accommodated my request, but even suggested a book and a course on fear of flying that was offered by a retired airline pilot. Ironically, the course being in another city meant she would have to overcome her fear of flying to take a course on overcoming fear of flying. The book was helpful.

While waiting for our flight at LAX, I tried hard to explain to Carol that this was the first time that I was not able to control my emotions. Later my daughter, enriched by her own experiences, would say, "By your age most people have already had a phobia. Now you understand my fear of flying." Indeed, The National Institute of Mental Health's research shows that 6.5% of Americans have a specific phobia, such as aviophobia, the fear of flying. This phobia has been described as having a "claustrophobia about being trapped in a thin tube" (My Age of Anxiety, Scott Stossel), which certainly had been true for me. One of the side benefits of heart surgery was that it enabled me to better understand that at times emotions can overrun rationality.

On our flight from L.A. to Dallas I learned that after the announcement on the previous flight "opened the bottle" for my new found phobia to come out, it was difficult to put back into the bottle. As the plane ascended, my mind raced with thoughts like "we are tilting approximately 30 degrees and it takes a speed of at least 150 miles an hour to keep us airborne. Given this, I estimate that we are going 200 miles an hour and still accelerating; so we must be passing 4,000 feet." My tried and true efforts at distraction would not work. I was mentally timing the flight. I was rational enough to recognize that my calculations were bizarre; but so emotionally removed that I did not care. I relaxed a little when I could breathe at my estimated 10,000 feet, the altitude at which the air pressure in the plane was set. But like any good engineer, I did not really relax until we added a safety factor of another 2,000 feet. What a lesson in the power of phobias.

At the airport in New York, we went in search of our luggage. What a surprise when we entered the luggage area just as the conveyor belt was delivering our bags from our original flight. All the time we spent involving a Dallas layover would have been spent on the tarmac. Was the Santa Barbara fog an omen?

New York: The next morning after months of being treated like a patient, I was treated as an equal by the people in the breakfast meeting of the CAB: I loved it. The high I felt when leaving the meeting was dealt a reality check when I was winded in my attempt to replace my previous jogs around Central Park with a walk around a single block or even crossing the busy street to see Madison Square Garden. This time there would be no jogs, no long walks around Times Square or Jackson

Square, no exploring the museums, no anything that required physical exertion. As I sat in the lobby an executive that I had career counseled pro bono stopped by to update me on his progress. This helped me understand that some aspects of physical progress would be slower than some mental ones.

During a delightful dinner, the president of this division of Mellon, whom I knew, sought me out and initiated a professional discussion. This was just the start of an evening that included many opportunities to remember how stimulating it was to share thoughts on an equal basis. What a lesson in balancing my physical recovery with social and business recognition.

That evening gave me the confidence to overcome my concern that if I accepted a long standing invitation for lunch with the President of the American Society of Corporate Secretaries, I could not hold up my end of the conversation. So I accepted his gracious invitation for lunch. I have found that by beginning with stating my concerns, such as not being fully recovered, reduces my stress levels, which it did. This may have influenced his steering our conversation towards the impact on our lives of our legal profession. It was fun. But it also illustrated that even, or maybe especially, in New York there were people who woke full of hopes, dreams and fears before hiding them underneath the dark business suits and picking up their briefcases that were full of the hopes, dreams and fears of others and, once again, seek a way to satisfy both.

These types of thoughts not only made staying true to myself easy, but as I walked by the Algonquin Hotel helped shift my memories from the business meetings in the hotel to the time I offered to take my daughter to New York for her first "legal" drink on her 21st birthday at the appropriately named 21 Club. The few friends she was permitted to bring morphed into my hosting seventeen twenty something year olds on her birthday, which happened to also be New Year's Eve. These brought the laughs, that after thinking of my memories of 9/11 converted to tears.

Fears: While sitting in the airplane at LAX my fear of the threat, real or otherwise, to my safety overwhelmed any other needs. Fears, or apprehensions, anxieties or concerns, are a real part of life that each of us must learn how to manage. My search for an example of someone when faced with physical threat who had managed to still consider other aspects of life led to the sports world. Jim Valvano, the basketball coach of North Carolina State, whose cancer had reached the point where he struggled to walk to the stage to deliver a speech at the ESPY Awards in 1993. He concluded with "If you laugh, think and cry, that's a full day." He closed by saying "cancer can take away all my physical abilities. It cannot touch my heart, it cannot touch my mind and it cannot touch my soul." No one has ever said it better. At some point, our hearts and minds become keys to recovery.

Exiting June: As I exited June, I reflected at how timely my trip to New York had been in contributing towards my rehabilitation. What a sequence! My rehab had provided an environment for discovering the internal and external beauty in my reduced world. Las Vegas had offered the greatest set of entertainment challenges man could design, and New York offered more of the same in the financial center of not only the U.S., but the world. The times were not always easy, but having my values tested by going from my small world of rehab to the fun, then business capitols of not only my country, but the world, was a terrific endorsement of my approach that I would like to share with others: this was the incubation of the idea for this book.

First satisfy major physical needs, then safety and security ones before social ones. Hope and a daily message was offered by Coach Valvano of "laughing, thinking and crying" (meaning be emotionally involved) by saying cancer (or heart problems) could take away his physical abilities but could not touch his heart, mind or soul.

Lessons learned:

1. Recovery from multiple heart surgeries takes time and patience. Expect many peaks and valleys along the way. Obtaining medical clearance, as I should have done before flying, can greatly assist the emotional aspects of managing perceived fears. Your behavior may appear irrational, and it may well be, but it will return to normal.

3. Successfully overcoming our fears, as will undoubtedly be less than the Coach's, is a huge step towards independence. People with restrictions, such as handicaps, can serve as role models for courage.

CHAPTER 22. INDEPENDENCE DAY

After the past few months of first having the opportunity to learn from my small world of rehab to appreciate some of the internal and external beauty that surrounded me, followed by challenging issues to have fun in Las Vegas and New York was a unique therapy. Would this July be the time I could join my country in celebrating our independences?

My earliest memories of my country's celebrations started as a child waving red, white and blue crape paper streamers through the wheels of first mine, then my children's, bicycle(s), for the 4th of July parade. So much fun, so much history, so much symbolism! The trumpets and drums of the high school band announcing the arrival of the proud faces of the bicyclist always caused the parents to clap and follow the parade through the historically preserved Haddonfield, New Jersey, which had been founded in 1701, down past the Haddon Fire Company (founded in 1764) and the Indian King Tavern, where the New Jersey Assembly met while fleeing the British in 1777 and which became part of the "underground railroad" used to hide fleeing slaves. Where but in America could a town celebrate its independence from a king on Kings Highway?

Thinking like a lawyer: I vividly remember the July day when I returned from attending a six-week Office of Civil Defense course on designing fallout shelters, when the radio proclaimed that the first man was walking on the moon. I interpreted this as encouraging citizens of this country to dream big: it was at that moment that I decided to attend law school. After graduating and becoming a Philadelphia lawyer, one of my favorite Sunday activities was to ride a bike to Independence Hall, where the First Continental Congress met and passed the Declaration of Independence; to the cracked Liberty Bell which rung to celebrate the signing; and then up to the Ben Franklin Parkway to the Philadelphia Art Museum for a jog up the steps made famous by the Rocky movies.

Now in this July after a successful surgery, stress test and trips to Vegas and New York, I did not anticipate any further impediments to my "Managing Your (my) Rehabilitation Program to WELL."

However, the exceptions started innocuously as Carol, returning from work, handed me a form while saying, "You are the lawyer. What do you think?"

My smile at being asked for a legal opinion for the first time since my surgery quickly faded as I said, "This is a form for you to apply for Voluntary Family Medical Leave. Are you applying?"

"No, of course not. I have to keep working for us to survive. Besides the bank needs me to continue my being Corporate Secretary and working with the board of directors, where the confidentiality requirements make it impossible to hire a temp."

"Why did they send it to you?"

"A woman in human resources noticed that I do not have regular hours in the office, even though my secretary has covered for me, and she decided I must take a family medical leave. But I have an agreement with the Chairman that I can work at home when necessary."

"I am surprised that she would send this to a member of the Chairman's office without first talking to him, or you."

"So am I," she said in a voice that meant that at this time she could not deal with the stress.

To reduce the stress, I said, "Since a voluntary program requires that you volunteer, and you haven't, the employee will quickly realize her actions violate the law, so simply ignore her."

Thinking we had just solved any potential disruptions to our safety and security, we turned to converting our unusable loft into an office that would be a designated place for my renewing my investing. To save time and money we hired a friend's husband, who besides his job writing manuals for a large aerospace contractor, had some experience in the construction business. This may have been a good idea at the wrong time, as my rehab had not progressed to where I could manage a good guy who was used to a budget of an aerospace company. He refused to submit a budget and when I drafted one, he both agreed and immediately ignored it.

While I was trying to control our spending, our income was again threatened when Carol handed me another copy of the same form she received in the mailed that was causing her so much stress! Disappointed because this rogue employee continued the error of her ways and surprised that she was unnecessarily increasing the stress on an already vulnerable Carol. In my human resources hat, I said, "This program is governed by a federal law that requires that they offer this type of program only on a voluntary basis. Send an email to this employee informing her that you have not, and will not, volunteer. Certainly she will have to honor a memo from the Corporate Secretary."

Thinking this solved that problem, Carol focused on her job and I on my attempts to limit the increasing expenses of the loft project by agreeing with every design. For example, the morning after Carol and I had spent hours studying the hundred pages of molding choices he had supplied, he installed his choice without even asking about our choice. I don't know which was worse: my frustration or having to listen to Carol's daily budgetary frustrations.

Then the fulcrum on which this set of stresses was balanced crashed when a teary eyed Carol handed me a form stating that she was being placed on unpaid "voluntary" family medical leave with the words, "You are the lawyer: handle it."

I felt my neck get warm as the blood rushed to my head. In my over thirty years in representing human resources departments, I had never seen this type of action. I knew better than to ask "why," or even "how," this employee could take this type of action without contacting Carol or the Chairman. When I put on my lawyer's hat and started working on our plan, my role shifted from receiving care to giving it to being a caregiver. A caregiver that wanted to protect my wife from unnecessary stresses as well as both of us from being in harm's way.

The lawyer in me organized our legal strategy. The issues were important to us and so far our non-confrontational attempts at resolving them had failed. I reviewed our potential ligation strategy. If we filed a complaint, these would be theories, or "counts," to pursue:

Count 1: Violations of the "Voluntary" Family Medical Leave Act by eliminating the voluntary aspects,

Count 2: Violations of the federal Fair Labor Standards Act, aka the "Wage and Hour" law, by "suffering or permitting" (the operative words), an employee to work, even at home, without compensation,

Count 3: Violations of the California Department of Industrial Relations for suffering or permitting work without pay.

Count 4: Violations of the employment contract with the Chairman that provided that she could work at home.

In my role as husband, I wanted to strike back at the cause of all the unnecessary stress that was hurting my wife! However, my experience in managing hundreds of lawsuits was that, win or lose, they always caused stress and permanently changed relationships. So how to immediately stop this renegade action that threatened our security and safety without damaging Carol's longer term relationships? To be sure congenial relationships were important for the trust necessary to be effective. What should we do?

Our last non-confrontational resort had to involve the Chairman. However, if I, as an attorney, had that conversation, I felt it would be disempowering to Carol as a person and a woman. So I said, "Advise the Chairman and if there is not an immediate response, I'll file the papers."

The Chairman took prompt action that even this employee could not ignore. Carol's compensation was "re-established," there was no break in our medical coverage and all the relationships were preserved. I wondered how an employee who was not married to an attorney, or worked for the Chairman, would have fared?

Work days: After the threat of losing our income, we reduced our expenses by finishing the loft project ourselves. Our days then began with a 6 A.M. wake up call, which was not the sound of soft music or even an alarm clock, but the beep, beep from her Blackberry since she turned it off at 11 PM. Who, I would ask, was sending you messages between those hours since your bank only operates in this time zone? The problem was that her bank was experiencing increased pressure from regulators and a takeover attempt. When the only solution was for her to work harder and longer, I saw in her the same symptoms I had experienced 25 years ago, about the time my arteries started to clog, while working and caring for a sick spouse. For periods I would be in denial; other times the stresses and weariness would be so strong that my shoulders and back would ache. Now I saw some of the same physical symptoms of weariness in Carol as she was fighting a flair up of her carpal tunnel syndrome, for which the only remedy was the impossible one of not typing. Her voice would say, "I'm fine," while her eyes and posture denied it, and she would inadvertently grunt when she got onto the sofa and reached for her laptop and cell phone.

Later when Carol was speaking at a conference of the Society of Corporate Secretaries, I got a glimpse of the stresses she had been under. Her response to the question of "How many sets of minutes do you write in a year" of 96 made the audience gasp: the audience averaged 12 sets.

Independence: Our evenings and weekends became extensions of the work days as we finished the mahogany wood surfaces of our loft project. I was too unsteady to work from the two-story ladder so Carol finished the sanding and varnishing of the wood.

I entered July thinking I could avoid challenges to my values by staying home. However, I was forgetting the warning of the book title "The Enemy Within," (Kris Lundgaard (1998),) or for Carol, in the bank, the words of Michael Corleone "Keep your friend close and your enemies closer" (the movie the Godfather part II). Entering July had provided my country and me to be reminded by the spirit of the 4th of July that some freedoms are worth the fight!

Lessons Learned:

1. Protecting security and safety needs from the threat of losing the financial means to pay for the security needs of housing, food and medical care is necessary to ensure our physical needs.

2. Sometimes there are positive aspects to an otherwise negative event; the threat to Carol's salary and benefits enabled me to improve my feelings of self worth by becoming a caregiver.

CHAPTER 23. AUGUST: FIGHT OR FLIGHT?

August brought with it my expectations that the events of May, June and July had provided an opportunity for me to master all the possible challenges to my physical, safety, security, and social needs. The events of August would show why I was wrong!

My now regular beach walks were helping to increase my stamina with a reasonable expectation that my improvements this time would be permanent. I was pleased to have solved a legal matter important to our survival and now looked forward to using my new loft to re-enter the ever challenging investment world demonstrated by the Money Show. This was a good time to start since the pace of the investment world slowed in August as many of New York's key players spent time in the Hamptons on the eastern shore of Long Island. The pace of the entire business world also slowed, although not as dramatically as the almost stop that annually occurred in Paris, as well as the rest of Europe. Locally, when there was a slight pause in the forces on Carol, and her bank, she asked, "I need a break and we have a week's timeshare that will expire this month. How about a quick trip to Mexico? The only resort available at this late date is in Mazatlan."

Mazatlan: "Sure," I said, hoping my words sounded more enthusiastic than I felt about leaving my new loft and now daily beach walks on the dog friendly Hendry's Beach. Deciding that there was virtually no risk of encountering any more stress at a Mexican beach than a California one, I reluctantly agreed to help Carol get away. So I said,

"Mazatlan sounds ok," completely unaware that just six months prior the U.S. State Department had issued a statement about Mazatlan: "Prone to petty crimes, like robbery and muggings." (February 5, 2007).

I gambled that the circumstances that had stoked my recent fear of flying would not be repeated; and they were not, although you can imagine my relief when we landed! The Mazatlan airport was as crowded as expected. Enthusiastic "entrepreneurs" were trying to crowd us into slowing down so they could describe all the wonders that they, and only they, could offer us; like wonderful taxis, fishing and timeshares. My recent experiences had increased my appreciation of people trying to earn a living, instead of begging, so I smiled and said "no gracious" to each offer. The van an airline employee recommended traveled past dirt fields with crumbling, unoccupied industrial buildings scattered among small adobe buildings with steel rods sticking out as though they were not yet completed. I later learned that the incomplete look was intentional because once they appeared finished, their taxes would be increased. The objective was to be fully functional while appearing incomplete. What a great example refuting the argument that higher taxes do not influence people's behavior. Adapting in Mazatlan was a way of life for the half a million residents of this commercial seaport on the Sea of Cortez.

The road dead-ended into choices of turning left leading to a long empty causeway along an empty beach, or to the right on a road running parallel to the sea with a few buildings on the left side. We turned right and continued for about a mile to our destination, the tallest building at 26 stories: El Cid. Unlike the one at the airport, this lobby was almost deserted. We were delighted to have our choice of rooms and selected a unit on the 24th floor with a view of the Sea of Cortez. Our short walk to the elevators was skillfully blocked by a woman with a clip board trying to sell us another timeshare. Before my surgeries, I would have said something negative that would have caused her to give us a wide swath. But my months of being vulnerable had demonstrated how hard earning a living could be, so I said, "We have only just arrived." As I would painfully learn, she heard these words as "there is hope so try again later."

There were three all glass elevators and one with solid walls. Since we were both a bit claustrophobic, we took a glass one. As it passed through the three-story high ceiling of the lobby, we were pleasantly surprised to learn that by running up the outside of the building, they provided terrific views of the surrounding areas. Our unit was on the corner with extensive windows on two sides providing panoramic views of the ocean and shoreline to the south. That night the windows rattling and the building shaking explained why we had our choice of rooms: it was hurricane season. However, the next morning the sun pouring in those same windows provided panorama views of the water and the squawking of the circling seagulls whose preference for the 24th floor would remain one of nature's charming unknowns.

We settled into a routine of a quick breakfast, a glass elevator trip down, a "no thanks" to the timeshare lady as we exited for our walks before the heat of the day. Unlike the resorts we had visited in Cabo San Lucas and Puerto Vallarta, this one was not self contained and the beaches were too steep, so we reluctantly chose the broken cement sidewalks towards the circle we had passed in the van. The sea side of the road was developed and reasonably well maintained. The other side was littered with small, poorly maintained businesses, some of which were still open. Earning a living in Mazatlan did not appear to be easy. My slow, tentative steps over and around the breaks in the sidewalk were clear indications that I was still pretty feeble. Our afternoons at the pool were restfully filled with reading mindless novels in the farthest corner from the loud speakers and the bar. It seems tourist have trained the hospitality personnel that all Americans want loud music to accompany fruity cocktails. In the evenings, wine accompanied quiet, relaxed dinners provided just the right slow pace. It was wonderful to see Carol's worry lines replaced by laughter as we reproved the adage, or at least it should be an adage, that reducing stress can re-stimulate marital interest just as quickly as increasing it can kill it.

A boardwalk: My experiences were that boardwalks meant multitudes of people walking, riding amusements and entering stores. Wednesday, we decided to extend our walk past the circle and learned that what was euphemistically called a "boardwalk" in Mazatlan was a long, empty, six-mile stretch of concrete causeway. "Multitudes" of people meant us; the only "amusements" was the large empty beach on our right that led to the Sea of Cortez; the only "stores" were the few deserted buildings with doors sealed by wooden panels decorated with graffiti on the other side of the street separated by vast amounts of dirt. There was nothing living: no people, dogs, trees, bushes, grass or even weeds. The only movement separating this street from a ghost town was an occasional passing farm truck. My travels had taught me to always be aware of my surroundings, so after walking a slow, unsteady mile, I glanced over my shoulder as movement caught my eye. Now there was a person where just a minute ago there had not been. Isn't that unusual, I thought, that suddenly, this person was about two hundred feet behind us on this causeway to nowhere in this town where all week we had not seen another walker. To test whether this was a coincidence or a reason for concern, I surprised Carol by stopping and turning sideways pretending a sudden interest in the deserted sand and sea while my peripheral vision scoped out that person who also stopped. It seemed highly unlikely that he had suddenly developed the same interest.

His looking at the sea provided an opportunity to see that this strong looking guy appeared to be twenty-something. He appeared to be a local; we did not. I was taller and paler than the residents, and my shorts, tee shirt and baseball cap shouted tourist. Carol was also too tall, blond, pale and was dressed in attention attracting shorts. As we turned to continue, my concern increased when I could not see anyone else.

We continued our very slow, tentative steps. While pretending to be talking to Carol, I glanced backwards and saw that he was walking as slow as we were. My antennas went up. It was humbling to know that I would not be able to protect Carol or, for that matter, even myself. I said, "Carol don't make it obvious but I think the man is following us. Let's find out." We stopped. He stopped.

We started walking a little faster: and so did he. My test had eliminated any doubts about whether this was an unlikely coincidence or a cause for concern. My mind started racing. I felt if we showed any interest or fear, it might cause him to immediately act. His maintaining a constant distance indicated to me that he was waiting for the right time and place to act. Hoping for help, I scanned the few buildings on the other side of the street hoping to find one that was not boarded up: no luck. Nothing, not even a stray cat or dog, was moving: except the guy following us.

I quickly reviewed our alternatives. Any attempts at fight or flight would be useless. Even if he were not armed, and with his intent he almost certainly would have at least a knife, in my condition I could not out fight him. Attempts at flight in my condition of having trouble even walking, would also be unsuccessful.

What about help? A quick glance of our side of the street showed only sand, and the other side only had dirt interspersed with graffiti laded boards over doors and windows. The only person remotely in sight was the driver of a stopped taxi on the other side of the street over a half a mile away. Any external help was highly unlikely.

What about internal help? Could I out think him? I doubted that I could think our way out of this crisis. But whether I could buy time was racing through my mind when I saw that we were entering an area where, if I were a predator, I would choose to strike. Our time was up. His closing the distance between us indicated that he had the same idea. Our time was up: it was either fight or flight.

"Carol, don't hesitate or question what I say. Just do as I do," I whispered as I turned, took Carol's hand and, drawing on all my adrenaline, threw my shoulders back to look threatening while walking as fast as I could back towards him. If we were successful, we would disrupt the timing of his plan. If we were unsuccessful, by closing the distance, we were decreasing our chances. I was banking on his fear of the unknown being greater than his fear of the known, so to shift his thinking from our vulnerability to his own, I aimed my left shoulder directly at his right shoulder. I avoided eye contact but my peripheral vision showed his eyes widening and his entire demeanor twitch. His freezing caused me to brace and prepare to deliver a shoulder-forearm smash, like I used to do to potential tacklers in football, before he took an unsteady step to his right. We passed close enough to smell his surprise. I had bought a little time: now what?

My backward glance was returned by his confused look turning to anger as he realized that he had been tricked. His body stiffened and he started to follow us at a pace much faster than ours. His determined facial expression and posture shouted his purpose. I knew our time was now even shorter. I could not even maintain this pace let alone walk any faster. Again, we faced the fight or flight options against a now angry adversary. But in the few minutes of my plan, the taxi had started moving slowly, very slowly, and was still several blocks away. It was a long shot and the driver undoubtedly would not offer much help against an armed local: but it was our only shot.

Timing was crucial. If we waited here just a few more minutes the angry bandito would have us. If we crossed the street too soon, he could grab us over there. Even if we made the taxi, he could pull us out the opened sided taxi, which locals call "pulmonias." The driver could not be counted on for help, so it appeared our choices were fight here or cross the street and fight there.

When I heard heavy breathing, I whispered to Carol, "Do not hesitate." My spinning around in a way indicating that I was going to attack, caused his facial muscles to shift from anger to confusion and his feet to stop. Immediately I grabbed Carol's hand and said "Come on," while pulling her in front of the first of a series of farm trucks I had spied when they were a block away. I saw the driver's eyes widen as he hit his brakes to slow down to avoid us before continuing on his way.

My glance showed the bandito waiting for an opening in the series of trucks. Our only chance, the taxi driver, did not appear to see my waving so I gambled and stepped in the street right in front of his taxi. He rocked to a stop. As he was starting to follow the local custom of negotiating the fare, we climbed into his open sided pulmonia and said "go." Half expecting to feel a hand grabbing my shoulder, I turned to see the guy still trying to dodge the trucks to cross the street. Slowly, painfully slowly, as pulmonias are not built for speed, we pulled away, and I made my final eye contact with his hateful stare. Later, I would learn of the State Department's warnings to tourists about robberies, muggings and fatalities that caused cruise ships to cancel stops in Mazatlan (Fox News, Jan. 27, 2010) even before the 300 homicides gave it the third highest homicide rate in Mexico (USA Today, Feb. 21, 2012).

An elevator: The rest of our week was spent enjoying the sun and each other. Early Friday afternoon when the wind brought in clouds, we hustled from the pool. In order to avoid the now desperate timeshare lady, we varied our routine of waiting for a glass elevator and took the first available one, which was the enclosed one. After the glass elevators, we felt like we in a moving closet. We exchanged small talk while gliding upwards towards the 24th floor until, suddenly, without warning, we bounced to a stop. The dim overhead light went out. The control panel's lights went out. The doors would not open. Our fast breathing was the only sound interrupting the dark silence. I chose not to share my suddenly ominous visualization of us being suspended on the side of a building at what I estimated to be the twentieth floor. First Carol, and then me, groped for the control panel and pushed every button: nothing. I ran my hands over every inch of the front wall searching for a phone: there was none. I put my hand over my heart to try to monitor my now racing heart rate. I silently told myself that I must avoid stress. While I am not fond of heights, Carol is claustrophobic and uncomfortable in total darkness. She started to scream.

I took a deep breath and searched for a solution. I tried visualizing how the mechanics of an elevator would work. I felt certain American elevators, which always seem to be Otis elevators, would have a safety devise of a locking system to prevent a free fall. But was this one manufactured by Otis? I quickly factored in that all mechanical systems require maintenance; but not all of them get serviced regularly. I recalled recently noticing that the inspection sticker in the elevator in our condo building in Santa Barbara was two years out of date. What are the chances that one in El Cid, Mazatlan, was up to date?

Were safety devises dependent on power? How wide spread was the power outage? If our elevator was broken, then all bets were off on safety devises working in a broken elevator. I decided not to share my analysis with Carol. It was becoming more difficult to breathe. Was there any action we could take? Carol took action. I heard, but couldn't see, her drop to the floor while continuing to scream. I remembered the time of my free fall in the elevator in the law library of Rutgers University in Camden. Hitting the spring in the bottom of the shaft was a jolt even after dropping only one story: how about twenty? I was still visualizing this unshared thought when through the closed doors we heard voices speaking Spanish. I exhausted my Spanish by saying "*Buenos dais.*" Darn, I wished I had studied Spanish harder in high school. Carol started yelling in English, and the men seemed to get the message as we heard them trying to pry the doors open. I couldn't see my watch to time my heart rate, but I knew it was high. I decided to violate my doctor's warnings that straining my chest might break the surgical staples holding my ribs together, and did exactly the worst possible motion. I put one hand on each side of the shut inner doors and tried hard to pull them apart. Ignoring the burning in my chest, I managed to separate them by about two feet. A little light entered enabling us to see something moving between the still closed outer doors. There was hope. Then I got a closer look at the tip of the tool the workmen were using to try to pry the doors apart: it was a butter knife. After a minute the knife disappeared along with the voices. Silence can be so ominous. I wondered how long we could continue to dangle versus how long it would take, if the power was out in all the elevators, for these guys to prioritize us and walk down and back up twenty odd flights of stairs.

After what seemed like an hour, but was probably only around fifteen minutes, the burning in my chest forced me to release the doors and they slammed shut. Complete darkness again punctuated only by Carol's screams. We descended a few feet before an abrupt stop. Then a few jerky feet upwards and bouncing to a stop before again descending down a few feet. My thoughts that our elevator was out of control were interrupted by another jerky move upward. None of these moves could possibly be by design. We were out of control, which was confirmed by our now very slow, uneven pace upwards indicating that we were not being held up by any locking system. Again forcing the inside doors open, I held them with my elbows while I grabbed and pulled at the closed outer doors of a floor we were slowly passing by. I estimated that we were getting close to the top where there must be a release that permitted the elevator to descend: although this time in free fall. As we continued our erratic trip upwards, I felt any opportunities would be short. I said to Carol, "Get up and get ready to get off quickly." There was no response. I continued holding the inner doors open with my elbows while grabbing at the next set of outer doors passing by.

Suddenly these outer doors opened. We were two feet above a floor and still moving slowly up. I looked up. The bottom of the next floor looked awfully close and getting closer. If we got half way out and the elevator speeded up, we would be crushed against the next floor. If we delayed for even a few seconds, our exit would be blocked. We had to act quickly. "Get up and jump," I yelled. Carol did not move. We could not waste this chance. We did not have time for a discussion. "Get up and jump," I yelled with more force. This was the chance I had hoped for when I asked her to stand up. She was still on the floor. If I let go of the doors to help her up, our moment would be lost. We couldn't wait. I knew there were no words to quickly motivate her in her current state. What to do? I didn't want to leave her. I hoped and prayed that her primary fear was being alone. I said, "We are passing the 25th floor. I am jumping. Get up and follow me or be alone." Carol's response showed me she was hysterical and would not listen to reason. I pushed the doors open as wide as I could, ducked my head to avoid the now close next floor and jumped. I hit the floor and took two stumbling steps away from the door to give Carol room to land, if she followed me. She did. I grabbed her and we hugged, and hugged, and hugged. Then we breathed and walked down the one flight of darken stairs to our floor. We later learned that there was virtually no chance of our being immediately rescued as the power was out for four hours in our part of town. It remains a mystery how, powerless, our elevator jerked up and down.

That night we laughed when, in the elevator, I yelled "Jump," Carol had responded "This is not our floor."

<u>Confidence</u>: We fell asleep only to wake, as we did our first morning, to the circling, squawking seagulls' reassurance that nature had not changed. But had a week with close encounters with recalcitrant people, places and things, changed me?

"Thinking like a lawyer" led to a "yes and no" answer. "Yes" it proved the error in my thinking that I had faced all the possible challenges from people, places and things. "No" because I had withstood the challenges while also protecting my wife.

On the return van ride, I noticed my mistake in judging the strengths of the crumbling buildings solely by their weak looking exteriors: this was the same mistake made by the bandito. Thanks, Mazatlan, for the confidence of our knowing that we could successfully take responsibility for ourselves in a city designated so dangerous by the U.S. State Department that the travel ships would avoid it.

Lessons Learned:

1. Leaving our comfort zones, as well as our surroundings, is an important part of rehabilitation.

2. Being physically and emotionally able to function is an important first step in protecting ourselves.

CHAPTER 24. SEPTEMBER: A RETREAT

When this first September of my second life arrived, I could feel the building of optimism. Optimism for what might be the next step in what I now saw as a sequence of progressively more challenging events, identified by the month in which they occurred, were so effectively designed it was as if a therapist had designed them as an outline for managing your rehabilitation program.

My journey started with my hitting bottom, which is where many experts say all real changes must begin physically. The prolonged nature of my formal rehabilitation program enabled me to better understand myself and the beauty that was everywhere in my small world. To exit this small world, I had to learn to trust after a "lawyer like" cross examination in April. May offered an opportunity to confront a challenge to my safety and security followed by staying true to myself in the glitz and glitter of Las Vegas. June was learning how to handle a new phobia and the world's business capitol. July was another challenge to security extended to also protecting my wife. August was physical challenges from a person, place and thing to both myself and my wife. What would September bring?

<u>Transitions</u>: Starting on my first day of Kindergarten, Septembers had always meant transitions that included challenges. For example, just the day before Kindergarten my parents had brought home a Dalmatian puppy. The first time I held him was beside the lamp post by our house in Oaklyn, New Jersey. Oh the thrill of holding that six-week

old puppy! My choice of a name, Spot, took second place behind Gallant, after his award winning father. I still laugh when remembering my response to the teacher asking how many were in our family of "Does Gallant count?"

Transitions in Septembers became ingrained in my psychic during the twelve years in grades K-12 followed by another twelve in universities, where each September began with the optimism that this would be the academic year in which I would learn the tools to become a competent, decision-making professional. This would last until June when I would take any available work, from a paint factory to loading dock, to finance the next academic year.

On this first September of my new life, I could feel the building of the same type of optimism. Starting with the latest surgery, and hopefully last, I had met a variety of challenges from people, such as the bad guy in Mazatlan; places, such as being in an airplane; and things, such as elevators. Would September bring a transition?

My first hint was the innocuous sounding question Carol asked, "Would you like to spend a couple of days in Malibu? I am coordinating the bank's board of directors' retreat, which this year is in the conference center at Pepperdine University. I'll be in meetings all day so your days will be free."

After growing up in a small New Jersey town where we tried to spend some weekends in Ocean City, I surprised even myself by being reluctant to spend time in this place that had only been a magical name. But also I had enjoyed my time in business and I wanted Carol to enjoy hers, so I said, "I'd love to," while resolving to stay out of the way.

We took highway 101 south to Oxnard, then the scenic Pacific Coast Highway to the main campus of Pepperdine University. I doubt there is anyone who has ever driven this highway that hasn't had at least a passing thought of living on this coastline and perhaps even attending Pepperdine, whose campus stretches 830 acres down the side of a mountain to the Pacific Ocean. We drove up the ascending steep, well-groomed, grassy slopes hosting white stucco buildings with red tile roofs and tinted windows. At the top we found our destination, the Graziadio School of Business and Management. The views of the Pacific Ocean, Catalina Island and the Palos Verdes peninsula were spectacular. Its sheer beauty must have contributed to its attracting the high quality faculty and students that caused it to be ranked the second most popular business school in the country by U.S. News and World Reports.

Business retreats: The purpose of retreats is to stimulate a change---a reappraisal, shift, about-face in a person's or organization's ideas, opinions, or decisions, about how they behave or think about something (Thesaurus). For boards of directors it provided a setting for busy professionals to not be distracted by daily events so they could focus on the goals, strategies, and tactics of the organization. This location, or to think like a lawyer, this venue met these requirements and also provided an opportunity for the board, and some bank branches in the area, to interact.

I anticipated our room being one step removed from a monastery – was I ever wrong! As soon as I set our bags in our comfortable, stylish and well-equipped room, the board of directors, spouses, CEO, Carol, and I boarded a bus. So much for my staying out of the way! Our first stop was a new retail branch where the manager and his staff had their first opportunity to interact with the people who had the power to decide their fate. Their nervousness was palpable. Their adrenaline rush was contagious. I was subconsciously returning to my former role of evaluating people's speech and demeanor both in and out of courtrooms. I was again "thinking like a lawyer."

From there we visited a recently acquired high-flying financial advisory firm. The top rated advisor spoke to us in a polite, professional way. When I asked him about the framed shirt of a baseball player on his wall, his eyes sparkled when he said his dream of playing in the majors had been sidetracked by a knee injury. I instantly saw him as an example of someone who mid-career learned investing after his first career no longer offered him a secure future. Listening to him, and understanding the financial concepts, provided strong encouragement for expanding my fledging investing efforts. A somewhat subtle lesson I had been learning was that investing in stocks was investing in the future, and since this was always uncertain, investors had to have confidence in their abilities. Confidence tempered by hard work.

Our next stop was the Presidential Library of Ronald Reagan in Simi Valley. I had found it challenging to form and implement my values during times when so few agreed. I admired President Reagan's ability to accomplish this but, of course, at a much higher level. The organization of the library-museum traced his life. I knew that there were some similarities between the President and my stepfather, Charles Dixon Trombold. This walk, at this time in my rehabbing, enlightened me to some of the underlying values driving both of them. They knew each other as boys when trooping together through the woods around the namesake of Charles' middle name, Dixon, Illinois. Charles liked to relate the story of the time he pulled "Dutch," as he called Reagan, out of a river and built a fire to stave off the chill. Both did not deviate from their integrities, their *raison d'êtres*, of maintaining responsibility for themselves while also reaching out to help others. Both worked their way through college during the depression and then left the woods for careers: Reagan in movies and politics and Charles at Campbell's Soup. Both sought to help others become independent: Reagan as governor, then as president, when he, among other things, was instrumental in destroying the Berlin Wall. Charles, as his country's sole representative for the food industry to the United Nations World Food Council, where he tried to help the world learn to feed itself.

Both enjoyed keeping their fierce independence. Over dinner Charles casually mentioned that once when he was in San Francisco, he called the then Governor Reagan to see if he was available for dinner in an hour. After an aide said the Governor would be delighted to have dinner with him, Charles asked "Where?" The aide said in the governor's mansion, to which Charles said, "My invitation was for San Francisco. I am not going to Sacramento," and he didn't. Remaining true to their values, both these men later in life returned to the outdoors they cherished from their youth. Reagan built his rustic cabin on a pond in rural California: Charles built his on a pond he built in rural Virginia. Reagan cut fire wood to relax: Charles built log fences. Reagan rode horses around his ranch: Charles rode his favorite horse Tobey around his ranch tending to 200 cows and a few bulls. Reagan moved into town when he became too ill to handle the rural home: Charles moved to a lake house after becoming too ill at age 81 to handle his rural home. Both these men stayed true to their values while leaving their beloved rural area to provide for their families and contribute to the free enterprise system before returning to their "ranches." Both men did not feel restricted by the expectations of others, or their own past; if they wanted to do something, they did it. These men served as role models as I faced the inevitable challenges of trying to recreate myself, my values and "to thy own self be true" (Polonius speech in Hamlet, Shakespeare).

Our final stop before returning to the conference center was the casual reception on the veranda of a hotel. My understanding with Carol was that she deserved an opportunity to develop her own career. My role was as a guest. Since conversations tended to be different when a spouse was present, we would be careful to not spend too much time together. While this was established for her career, at this function it had another benefit. It forced me to interact with professionals I respected. The gracious reception of the others provided an environment in which I relaxed enough to have short, insightful conversations with bright people I barely knew. With each conversation, I could feel my confidence growing.

The next morning I hoped to quietly stay out of the way while partaking of the board's informal buffet breakfast. As I started for an empty table in the back w a full plate in hand, a board member said, "Brent, please join us." It seemed so natural to participate in a conversation with an attorney and CPA about a variety of economic topics. When a bell signaled the start of their meeting next door, I was alone. Alone, that is, except for the tray of Danish pastry. Not just any Danish, but my favorite, cherry, which were even better than the donuts that had pulled my steering wheel towards each Dunkin' Donut shop when I lived in New Jersey. Oh, I would tell myself that I was tired and needed coffee, which of course I could never have without a donut. Now in my second life, while I looking at the Danish the thought of my formerly clogged arteries filled my mind; so I refilled my coffee cup and walked out onto the veranda for a new day and a new life. Rehabilitating-to-recovery required some small changes in my habits, such as not thinking of donuts, as well as some large changes, such as not wondering whether my heart could handle any new activities.

As I walked out on that veranda the aspects of retreats became personal. My mind flashed back fourteen years to my first and only retreat, which was when I had turned fifty. After a couple of days of sitting by a pool looking at a blank legal pad, my retreat stimulated a change – reappraisal, shift, about-face – to thinking of myself as a business rather than as an employee. As a business, I needed a plan, so I started writing my first Annual Plan of goals and methods to accomplish them. My heart problems had caused me to drift from this year's plan that had been written just days before my heart stopped.

Now, standing alone on a veranda without any distractions, my subconscious utilized the power of suggestion of being at a retreat to stimulate "retreat like" thoughts. The setting could have been anywhere conducive to quiet introspection. I just happened to be sipping coffee while looking down over the campus to the ocean. Permitting my mind to wonder caused a change in perspective of the events of the last several months. So many of the events that had seemed so random could also be viewed as building blocks. I was learning the boundaries of my physical capabilities, how to slowly expand them and, hopefully, knowing when to stop, which I came to symbolize by the lyrics from a song of "know when to hold-um, know when to fold-um and know when to walk away." My trips served as benchmarks: Las Vegas dealing with social and business stimulation; New York with the same plus my life as an attorney; and Mazatlan with protecting not only myself, but Carol. When other people did not treat me as a heart patient: I had not acted like one.

Much like my past Septembers had brought first new teachers, then new universities, this retreat began with examples of the chairman and other board members making an "outsider" feel welcomed and valued; the financial guru demonstrating how to remember, but not dwell on, his first love of baseball; President Reagan demonstrating staying true to his values in so many different circumstance; as did Charles in his own way. So many examples that all it required was for me to be open to noticing, which was a major benefit of this retreat.

I knew that taking a "walk about" would permit my mind to constructively process my thoughts. As a humorous aside, I had raised many an eyebrow when, lost in thought and oblivious to my surroundings, I would walk around my office building moving my hands and muttering to myself. On this hilly campus, the only flat ground I could find was the university's track. After a short drive down the hill, I wondered about using the track when my breath quicken while just walking up the flights of steps from the parking lot to the track.

I took comfort that my Nike shorts, shirt and sneaks made me look like I was in the right place. However, I quickly proved how deceiving looks can be. When I started walking on the inside lane the dirty looks of runners reminded me that etiquette called for slower movers to move to an outside lane to make room for the faster ones. I was moving so slowly to the outside lane that I felt like the frog in the video game Frogger, who was trying to get through lines of traffic without being hit. From the outside lane, as I watched the runners, a strange thing happened: I missed jogging. Was that possible? What about it did I miss? Was it the feeling of accomplishment?

Without really thinking, I took a quick step with my right foot, followed by one with my left. This caused me to lurch unsteadily to my left. Automatically my right foot followed and brought me upright again. I was jogging; sort of. After twenty feet my breathing felt labored and I stopped and walked, while placing my hand over my heart. It was beating faster, but was that good or bad? A benefit of the rehab program was to learn to monitor myself. I could not identify any irregularity in my beats. What about the rest of me? Nothing was quivering, numb or hurt.

I decided to use this standard for physical activities to measure the impact after trying it as a replacement for the one used before the activity of "will it help, or hurt me." This willingness to try activities before judging them was a clear indicator of the transition from rehabbing-to-recovery that follows Managing Your Rehabilitation Program WELL:" hence the title of this book.

After forty feet, I put my right foot out quickly followed by my left and was jogging again; for twenty feet. Two college-aged joggers ran by looking as if they wanted to ask me if I was all right. I smiled as just like them, I was a jogger, just a slower one. I was no longer thinking like a patient: now there is a strong endorsement for retreat-type experiences.

To keep this exhilarating feeling growing, I needed a measurable goal with a timetable. Symbolically, my goal should be something I used to do, such as jog the three miles as I used to do by the Brandywine River, and the timetable should be on the first birthday of my second life. So that was it! To achieve this I needed a training schedule where jogging each day could be become a habit rather than a daily debate. For simplicity, my birthday was rounded to January 1. I needed the encouragement of achieving interim goals, which I selected to be to jog two miles on December 1, and one mile on November 1. To eliminate what jogging meant, I added that it had to be non-stop but, to reduce stress, did not designate a pace.

The audacity of my setting such goals when I could not jog 30 feet forced a laugh so loud that the runner passing me jerked her head towards me. I simply waved. I had transitioned from rehab to recovery. In that moment not much changed physically. Oh, I might have stood a little straighter, added a little bounce into my steps, and my jogging clothes might have felt like they fit a little better, but these were the effects, not the cause, which was the improvement in my "self-image."

My retreat: Unbeknownst by me at the time, standing on that veranda sipping coffee just after the others left to begin their retreat was also the beginning of mine. An advantage I had in assimilating where I was in my journey from rehabilitating-to-recovery was that each month had provided a different test of my physical and mental capabilities. My subconscious realized that month at a time, with some redundancies, I had successfully met every challenge by people, places and things to my capability to provide and protect my physical, safety, security and social needs, as well as maintaining a sense of self worth.

The impact of the assimilations of these was on the track with my transitioning to feeling like just another out-of-shape person. At lunch with my niece, Amy, I no longer felt any need to discuss me, so I directed the conversation to her plans and did the same thing that night at the board dinner. I hope the board's retreat was as successful for them as it was me.

Lessons Learned:

1. How you view yourself is powerful: it affects the way you act, which affects how others view you; which affects how you act. For example, the only time I called myself a heart patient was the time I wanted to get off the plane in LAX.

2. Other people's opinions can help to re-enforce, but not replace, your own. All real changes have to come from within.

3. While I was fortunate to have my retreat at Pepperdine, the same approach can be used in any venue that provides quiet solitude, such as a park, beach or mountain where reflection can lead to setting goals. Our environment can act as triggers for changes in our thoughts if we remain open to them.

CHAPTER 25. OCTOBER: VALUES AND HABITS

I entered October wondering how "Managing Your (my) Rehabilitation Program WELL" would help me give birth to a healthy lifestyle. To understand the application of concepts in my law practice, I had learned that it could be helpful to analyze the component words:

1."Managing" means having control or authority, as in administering, executing, governing or leading.

2. "Your or my" meaning the creator and owner of the program.

3. "Rehabilitation" means restoring someone or something back to a normal, healthy condition from an illness, injury addiction, as in recondition, renovate or revamp.

4. "Program" meaning a plan of things that are done in order to achieve a specific result or a set of instructions.

5. "Well" meaning the state of being happy, healthy and successful.

Using a technique of substituting synonyms could provide a sentence such as : "executing" "my" "restoring health" "to achieve" "being healthy." By using these words it is easier to identify that continuing the concepts of "Managing Your Rehabilitation Program WELL" was important since only "restoring" my health would restart the same cycle. An unintended result of searching for clarity was that the acronym for WELL" of "Will Enthusiastically Love Life" indicated that this program might also be useful for rehabilitating from other life threatening illnesses, injuries, addictions or imprisonment.

Birth month: For me, October represented the births of my sons, first Chad, then four years later Grant. There was a similarity in that their births, like mine this year, had been initiated nine months earlier by the activities of a couple of other humans. Of course, their "couple" had been their parents, and mine had been a vascular and cardiac surgeon whose efforts had made "One Heart—Two Lives" possible. In this October, I knew I had to change something in order to "give birth" to a healthy lifestyle.

A healthy lifestyle: When I asked my cardiologist how I could avoid future heart problems, his response of "lead a healthy lifestyle" was not a bad "opener" to use a poker term, but without more it was an "empty set" to use a mathematical term. My friends all said my habits were healthier than theirs, yet they were still standing. Same in rehab where I appeared to have the healthiest lifestyle and the worst medical condition. Any answers would have to come from within me.

Values: In summary form, this question began a very difficult introspection that led to my realizing that I had acquired many of my values from my father; such as, my word should be my bond, which to me included being honest with myself. Appreciate the rights of others, which may be one of the driving forces behind my becoming an attorney with a practice where I could enforce the fair and equal treatment for all employees. Never consciously hurt others, as illustrated by Google's motto of "Don't be evil." Help others through organizations, such as the YMCA, Opera Delaware and Mended Hearts.

At age sixteen, with the dreams of youth but without the guidance of maturity or a mentor, was a life changing moment when I learned the tough lesson that I could not rely on even my parents who, despite their promises, had not been saving for my education. I remember sitting in my room wondering that if I could not take the reassurances of my parents, then whose could I trust? From then on I learned to only depend on myself, which I rationalized with the thoughts that when humans were given the ability to think, it also included the duty to think. By thinking I could take responsibility for my actions.

In college I continued expressing my values through my habit of taking responsibility not only for selecting my courses, but also for what I studied within each course. When my professors disagreed, I never argued I just continued. A few professors reacted in non-professorial, personal ways. For example, one suspended me from class for violating having more than 4 cuts – I had 4 ½ – while I said the university policy provided suspension "on the 5th cut." He said I could not come back unless I could find an authority who supported my opinion. After the dean of the law school blasted him, the professor reluctantly readmitted me but lectured me on letting down my parents, my future children, the state and God! Imagine as a 20-year old being told by a professor of metallurgy that he was disappointing God! He was not the only professor with this attitude which contributed to my habit of paying less attention to opinions and more to their underlying reasoning.

Fortunately, not all professors shared this attitude and my habits facilitated my receiving a fabulous education while earning degrees in math, management, law and employment law. However, I now knew some of my habits may be problematic.

Habits: Activities that became "routine," as in "consistent, often unconscious patterns," were the words management guru Steven Covey used to define "habits." The power of habits had been known for centuries. In the words of Aristotle (384-322 B.C.), "Good habits formed at youth make all the differences." Habits are "something a person does often in a regular and repeated way" (Merriam-Webster).

I related to the three components of every habit being: (1) a cue that acts as a trigger, (2) the behavior, and (3) the reward (Charles Hopkins). At sixteen my "cue" was learning that to achieve my dreams, I was on my own; my "behavior" would be to be dedicated to obtaining an education; and my "reward" would be my lifestyle. Developing these habits contributed to my successes. However, if all my habits had a good long-term effect, then I would not be a heart patient. One habit I now knew I had to change was my requiring perfection in every activity. In trying to change this and other habits, I would learn the wisdom of Ben Franklin's words, "It is easier to prevent bad habits than it is to break them."

Stress as a habit: When my heart stopped, I had none of the causes that are generally assigned to heart failure – diet, exercise, weight, cholesterol and smoking – except for stress. And I knew I had a problem with stress. Yet stress was a natural part of life. I agreed that at times I may have had more than most. Besides losing my habit of requiring perfection for every activity, I also sought ways to improve the way I dealt with stress. I knew one way was to use what I called "stress relievers," which was the method that I felt helped me avoid the heart attacks of the other two executives who were under the same stress.

Establishing goals, as I did for jogging a mile on the beach by November 1, forced me to regularly overcome all the "too" reasons – I was too tired, or it was too hot, chilly or windy – by making it a habit.

A habit that included stopping at the top of the seven wooden steps to appreciate and give thanks for the sky, ocean and sand. My start of 500 (I have a habit of counting things) slow, unsteady steps to reach the marker of a gate at the bottom of a path down the cliffs gradually became a milestone on my way to taking 1,300 steps to the large rock sticking up out of the sand. Touching that rock provided a thrill that I had not gotten from a rock since feeling the vibrations from a rock at Stonehenge, which still puzzled me: why did I feel the vibrations in a stationary rock, and why didn't everyone?

My heart problems required that I slow down, which offered opportunities for me to step away from the normal distractions and learn about my surroundings. I was slowly learning that during my rehabilitation, I had been "Using a limited environment to get in touch with the world" (Ralph Waldo Emerson). Looking back I realized that my lunch time jogs along the Brandywine River Valley in Wilmington, Delaware, had inspired an interest in that environment. Visits to the Brandywine River Museum had introduced me to a person with the same interest: the painter Andrew Wyeth. Andrew reduced his distractions by reducing his environment to summers in rural Maine and the rest of the year in the Brandywine River Valley, where he painted his intensely personal reactions of his relationship with surrounding objects, such as windows, barns, tree branches, and his neighbor Christina. Now I had a better understanding of why I was so attracted to his paintings. My new appreciation of the value of the introspection of Andrew's paintings led to an appreciation of Henry David Thoreau. Thoreau, to get better in touch with his surroundings, lived alone for two years in reduced surroundings next to a small pond. He emerged with a better understanding of himself that he wrote about in his classic book *Walden's Pond*.

While I certainly do not have the talent of either of these artists, in a metaphysical way I was also learning to appreciate the beauty that

Thoreau and Wyeth saw: and the stress just disappeared.

Now my jogs became fascinating learning experiences as Hendry's Beach provided my "window to the world" in much the same way Walden's Pond had for Thoreau and the Brandywine valley had for Wyatt. Sand was a home to many microorganisms that provided a food source for birds and small fish. The tides enabled the ocean to re-circulate some things, like kelp and drift wood. Kelp provided a home for sand fleas and other parts of the food chain, while also helping to prevent beach erosion. The drift wood raised thoughts of how it was used to build ships to carry people and cargo from one port to another. Rocks helped prevent the tides from sweeping away the sand and driftwood. On my jogs I began to see the similarities between nature, which used a predictable structure that, when destructive, had to be altered; and the same being true for my habits.

My goal of jogging a mile by November 1st was aided by my making jogging a habit. As a habit, when facing my feeble efforts, rather than consider quitting, I sought ways to improve. Instead of jogging until I felt tired, I alternated jogging and walking for twenty steps. What an amazing difference! By eliminating the habit of internally debating when to start and stop, the total distances greatly increased. Of course without my insisting on "doing it myself," I could have learned this phenomenon was called "interval training," but then would I have made it a habit?

Just a few days after celebrating my sons' birthdays, while dressing as a track star for Halloween, as the costumes of ghosts had become too personal, I noticed that my silhouette stood a little taller and straighter and my head no longer tilted forward.

Perhaps for the "thoughtful" person described by my surgeon, taking charge of your rehabilitation program might be slow but it also would lead to not only my returning to my previous mental and physical health, but to also improving them in a way that could help prevent restarting the heart disease cycle. Now that was a powerful set of reasons to continue "Managing Your (my) Rehabilitation Program WELL."

Lessons Learned:

1. The predictable steps in returning to an independent life style are satisfying our physical needs, than those for security, social interaction

and feelings of self worth. Some setbacks are to be expected and must be worked through. There is no timetable. Sometimes it will appear that there is no progress until an event illustrates the hidden progress.

2.The initial goal is to be able to independently function physically, mentally and emotionally. The risk of simply restoring yourself to the condition that you were in just prior to the discovery of your heart problems is that this condition (and those activities) had led to heart problems. Preventing this from occurring requires an analysis of your values and habits and then changing the destructive one(s).

This requires an introspection, which for me was difficult and time consuming. But the time I used was when my alternative activities were limited by my physical limitations. The positive is that the rewards can be life changing in the positive way. The mentioning of Wyeth, Thoreau and Emerson were meant to illustrate the awaking of a new perspective for appreciating my surroundings.

3. We all do pretty much the same things every day. To test your values and habits, try doing the same things differently and the reactions of others will assist you in understanding yourself.

5. There are lessons everywhere.

CHAPTER 26. NOVEMBER: GOAL SETTING

On Thursday, November 1, I arrived at the beach nervous. Would I regret the audacious goal made on the spur of a moment to jog a mile non-stop? My heart pounding always reminded me of my college roommate, the track star Steve, telling me, "You must relax when running to enable your chest to expand easier." My having a high level of stress was proof that relaxing was never easy for me. Remembering that recent years I had been given the same advice for golf. On this day, I took deep breaths while uttering a silent "thanks" towards the sky and the power that was responsible for creating the beautiful environment and permitting me to enjoy it. It helped.

I walked down the wooden steps to begin the warming up walk to the small rock where, out of habit, I started jogging. Indeed, relaxing was the key, so I shook my arms, rotated my neck, and step after step shifted my thoughts to the beauty of the beach. I had learned that focusing on long distance markers permitted my mind to start the "your legs are tired" game, so as silly as it might sound, my new habit was to select interim markers. Reaching each marker provided a feeling of "can do" as I set my sights on the next one. No long distances, just a compilation of short ones. Markers passed and my mind wondered with only one topic being off limits: thinking of stopping. Then I saw the marker for a mile. My emotions spiked. It was only two close markers away. Then one, then none! In my mind I heard the music from the movie Chariots of Fire, a film about the sacrifices made by two British sprinters to win Olympic medals. I raised my arms to break the imaginary tape as I crossed the imaginary finish line. I won! I met my first interim goal towards the three mile goal.

Why was jogging a mile so important to me? It was so much more than just a physical accomplishment. It was a triumph of using a goal to create a habit to support my value of taking responsibility for my health. I related to the saying, "A goal is a dream with a deadline" (Napoleon Hill). On that day, on the track, at the bank's retreat, the passing joggers stirred a vision of how satisfying jogging had been in my past. I agreed with the entrepreneur who said, "Visualization is critical." One amazing illustration of the power of visualization was the study that found that " the brain patterns activated in weightlifters when lifting hundreds of pounds of weights was similar to the patterns activated when they only imagined lifting" (Psychology Today). Motivational speaker Tony Robbins related visualization to goals with the words, "Visualization is the first step in turning the invisible into the visible."

A motivating force during my rehabilitating-to-recovery was visualizing myself as I was in my first life, but I realized I had to eliminate those habits that had caused my heart problems. The principles of "Managing Your (my) Rehabilitation Program WELL" had successfully accomplished two things: they enabled me to identify the interim goals of my physical, safety, security, social, and self worth needs, and then satisfying them in order to create a structure for my "One Heart—Two Lives" to be successful. But was this really a final goal, or just another interim goal?

Goals: A goal has been defined as "The object of a person's ambition or effort, an aim or desired result." A goal is a target, purpose, aspiration, dream – even a hope (Merriam-Webster).

Setting goals was not a new concept as many a New Year's Eve I joined the millions in pausing, perhaps with a celebratory glass in hand, to spontaneous make goals that we labeled "resolutions." Mine were as well intended and admirable as those identified in a study that showed that 86% of the people surveyed had their resolutions include "better health," 83% to "get in better shape," and 80% to be "happier." Yet despite great intentions, the pattern of their being violated by January 20 (IBD, 1/5/2007) indicated that they were really "hopes." Why?

I thought it might be that they were too general so I used "to do" lists. That is until the day I found a list from fifteen years prior that contained the same items as my current one: spend more time with family, make more money, exercise more. Like my goal of perfection, my goals lacked specifics. As early as the sixth century B.C., Confucius is quoted as saying, "When it becomes obvious that goals cannot be reached, don't adjust the goals, adjust the actions steps."

Goal setting: When I turned fifty I asked, "Where will I be in five, ten and fifteen years if I change nothing?"

Besides causing me to gasp, this question also changed my life! It led to my discovering two studies. The Yale study involved asking graduates from 1953-1973 for their goals as they graduated. The follow up showed that the 3% who had specific goals accumulated more wealth than the other 97% combined. The Harvard study asked graduating MBAs from 1979-1989 for their career goals:

--3% had written goals

--13% had goals but not in writing

--84% had no specific goals

The follow up years later showed that the 13% with non-written goals earned twice as much as the 84% without any goals. However, the 3% with clear, written goals were earning on average 10 times as much as the total of the other 97% combined.

Since all the students at these two universities had already met their relatively rigorous goal of admissions, the only reason I could attribute to the wide disparity in these results was written goals. The size of these studies indicated that, statistically, they were valid. Writing specific goals greatly increased the probability of achieving them – period! These results are indisputable.

As a younger man I might have made a mental note of these studies and immediately shifted to the needs of the moment. But at age fifty, the question of my future could no longer be put off until tomorrow. My experiences paralleled those of the Yale and Harvard studies. When I had specific goals, such as law school, and I visualized the results, like being a lawyer, I generally achieved them. My search for why this worked led me to concluding that it motivated my subconscious to search for ways to achieve these goals. It worked so well that I should use it for all my goals: but first I needed to define my goals.

I recommend creating your own "retreat like" environment,

meaning free of the normal distractions of life. As I sat by a motel pool, hundreds of miles from home, with only my trusted clipboard and grasped my felt-tipped pen, the blank page on my legal pad seemed to stare back with the question: Where to start?

I would have grabbed any available distraction: but there weren't any. I stood and circled the pool using my voice to stimulate my sense of talking and listening (this is best done when alone) searching for a place to start. Finally (duh) I started at the beginning. How did I want to visualize a typical day in 5-10-15 years? I saw a smiling, active person enjoying the physical recreation activity with his family. Ok, that was a start, now what were the components of this vision? "Being physically, financially, and emotionally able to lead an active life," which I wrote as my objective.

This objective made me feel good but even these feel good eleven words would not provide my subconscious with any way to visualize any necessary interim goals. I thought of this as being a lack of the specificity necessary to create interim goals that could cumulate into my objective. I needed to create annual plans.

We were successfully using annual plans at work, which we called an accountability system. So I decided to try it in my personal life. The system was each year to write a one page annual plan setting forth goals and, crucially, specific ways to achieve them. This solved the need for specificity, which enabled my subconscious to create implementation habits. Under each of the general topics – physical, financial, emotional and relationships – there would be specific goals for the year. My jogging will be used to illustrate the requirements for every goal:

1. Written.
2. Attainable, specific and measurable, for example "jog a mile" instead of "jog more."
3. Results oriented and active, for example "jog a mile" instead of "study whether to start jogging."
4. Have dates, for example "jog a mile by November 1.
5. Phrase positively, for example replace "I will run continuously," rather than, "I will not stop."
6. Each entry should be short and separate.

I am embarrassed to say that my annual plans worked so well that after I achieved all of my initial goals within five years, I became complacent, confident, pleased, satisfied and, dare I say, "smug."

My failure to continue to implement these plans was also sabotaged by my violating the anachronism KISS, Keep It Simple Stupid, is key. Over the years I had let my plans morph into containing too many topics to be effective. My plans that had started with 10-15 goals had grown into 46 in the plan written days before my heart stopped. I recommend between 10-20, and my new one had 17. I still considered it a "living" document in that it could be altered to comply with changing circumstances.

In the words of Thomas Jefferson, "Nothing can stop the man with the right mental attitude from achieving his goal; nothing on earth can help the man with the wrong mental attitude."

MAP: Now that "Managing Your (my) Rehabilitation Program WELL" had brought me close to rehabilitating-to-recovery, it was time to decide what was next? Previously when I stopped creating or implementing a plan, I had drifted into behavior that led to heart disease. Now that I was a heart patient, it was vitally important to avoid this type of behavior: but how?

Why not combine the principles of my successful "Managing Program" with those of annual plans in a program labeled "Managing Annual Plans," or the acronym MAP?

The interim goals under my "Managing Program" would be incorporated into annual goals under the MAP system, as indicated by the chart below that relates each step of one program to the corresponding step in the other program:

Steps	Managing Your Rehabilitation Program	Managing Annual Plans
1.	Physiological	Physical
2.	Safety and Security	Financial
3.	Social	Emotional, relationships Family
4.	Self Worth and Self Esteem	Achieved through the above Plus any miscellaneous items

The programs were startlingly similar! It would appear that "Managing Your Rehabilitation Program WELL" would transition smoothly into "managing Annual Plans" utilizing many of the same principles and lessons learned.

<u>Additional benefits</u>: I needed a stimulus for jogging that would reduce the stress by eliminating the debate and guilt associated with "excuses" for not exercising for at least the minimum half hour a day, five days a week, recommended by the medical community. During October through December my goal of jogging three miles on New Year's day had provided an interim goal for completing my rehabilitation. But I needed motivation to prevent my joining the 70% of post-surgical heart patients who would not be meeting the medical minimum exercise just nine months after their surgery. Since the 30% who still exercised was also the percentage of the general population who exercised, it appeared that having a heart attack did not stimulate most heart patients into changing their habits. Following a MAP would have many benefits.

I view MAP as having both physical and a mental aspects, which can be combined. I use my beach time as providing an opportunity to get in touch with my subconscious without any distraction. It turns out that these times provided an opportunity to learn the meaning of the saying, "The scenery, when it is truly seen, reacts on the life of the seer" (Ralph Waldo Emerson). Opening my eyes and mind to my surroundings opened me to seeing that "Every particular in nature, a leaf, a drop, a crystal, a moment in time is related to the whole, and partakes of the perfection of the whole" (Emerson). Rehabilitating had opened my receptivity; first for inanimate objects, like rocks, and then a new appreciation of life in simple things like sea shells. Now besides admiring their intricate beauty, I also thought of what an amazing process for small, soft creatures to create their own security system to protect them from the predators.

While jogging to overcome my disability, I began to notice the universal fight to overcome disabilities, such as the three-legged dog and the one-legged seagull trying to keep up, which reminded me of hobbling down hospital corridors flashing in my open gown. Seals offered many examples, such as the wounded seal trying to recover by hiding so well among piles of kelp that it took his snaring teeth to alert me that I was about to step on him, reminding me of my need for rest post lung surgery. Or the one searching for sufficient strength to defend itself from the attacking dog, reminding me of my searching for a weapon as I lay in post surgery listening to the demented attorney in the next bed. Or the one escaping back into the sea, reminding me of my 3 A.M. escape to another hospital room. Or the one climbing onto a rock to escape sharks reminding me of my "fight or flight" in Mazatlan. Sadly the remnants of a dead seal was a reminder to me of the importance of continuing to fight for life. We really are all in this together.

So many lessons offered on the security and social aspects of life, like the plover birds scrambling along in the surf trying to keep up with the pack, the dolphins taking turns breaking the surface as their pod swam close to shore, and the whales swimming in groups as they migrated back and forth served as reminders of my travels.

Dogs offered so much inspiration, such as their desire to protect their owners being so strong that, at times, they were almost choked by their own enthusiasm. When off lease, they ran ahead to scout the areas while continually checking back to be certain their owners were safe and secure. They paid special attention to owners who had physical disabilities, such as lack of mobility or sight, while trying to overcome their own, like the three-legged dog keeping up with his master. They demonstrated social caring by returning the balls and sticks their owners kept losing. Watching a beautiful, brown Great Dane encapsulated so many aspects of life in such a short time. I first saw him as frisky puppy not aware of his own size or strength. When he did puppy things, people and smaller dogs shied away. Watching him progress so quickly from a frisky puppy to a lumbering, frail animal was sad. Initially he had gracefully scampered up the steep slope to his home. In far too short a time, instinctively he seemed to understand that this was no longer a good idea so he ever more cautiously climbed. Finally he refused to try and relied on help from his master, much as I had in the hospital. Even other dogs sensed his weakness and some smaller dogs that had avoided him now sensed vulnerability and harassed him; reminding me of the bad guy on the causeway in Mazatlan.

Jogging had stimulated so much more than just physiological improvements. Besides feeling stronger and more secure in my movements, I felt more in touch with my surroundings and their interactions, which changed my attitude. Changing my occasional jogging to a habit had made a crucial difference by eliminating the "too" habit used by joggers and golfers: the day was too hot or cold; too wet or dry; the course was too hilly or flat; too rocky or sandy; and the player was always too busy, tired, sore, or stressed; and, well, you get the point. Making something a habit directed my subconscious away from this list and towards finding a way to jog in almost any setting, perhaps varying the length, timing or duration to accommodate almost any requirements; equipment simply required a little planning and flexibility.

MAP, by applying the lesson learned from the Yale and Harvard studies, would provide a systematic method of continuing to apply the successful principles of "Managing Your Rehabilitation Program WELL" towards achieving my goals of "Being able to physically, financially and emotionally lead an active life."

It has been said that "What you get by achieving your goals is not as important as what you become" (unknown). My feeling was that I did not volunteer for heart problems, but having had them I wanted to utilize the principle learned while rehabilitating-to-recovery to "become" the person I had long visualized.

This Thanksgiving I was thankful for a great number of things, starting with deep breaths.

Lessons Learned:

1.	Goals can be a motivator and, when written, can lead to some creating habits that improve our lives.
2.	Goal setting can be particularly helpful for our subconscious mind if the goals are clearly defined, attainable, measurable, and broken into interim steps.
3.	The same principles that made "managing Your Rehabilitation Program WELL" successful can be continued through "Managing Annual Plans," or MAP, successful.
4.	Even temporary changes in perspective can teach us a great deal as there are exciting lessons everywhere in the world, from which we can learn a great deal about ourselves while becoming the person we want to be.

CHAPTER 27. DECEMBER: WARNING SIGNS

The sun gleamed off the nervous sweat on the face of the man as he stepped out of his car. He was a man with a purpose. It was race day at Hendry's Beach, and he looked the part in his new black Nike shorts and red tee professionally designed to whisk away the anticipated sweat. The low white runners' socks highlighted new silver and black Saucony running shoes, selected for their high arches. The ball cap from one of his alma maters, the University of Tennessee, did not yet have sweat dripping off the visor. When he reached the top of the steps, his habits took over: pause and scan the horizon, take the steps down to the short walk in the warm sand to that certain rock, shake shoulders loose and quickly take a first step with left foot, then the right; repeating this pattern while getting acclimated with the sand and surf on the deserted beach. Jog to the big rock, then the blue house on the cliff with the little white dog before heading to the house on the top of a cliff where the Great Dane lived. He noticed that the flowers decorating the cliffs were an ever changing kaleidoscope of colors as first yellow, then red, sprung into dominance. He was learning to appreciate the lessons taught by nature, such as the cliffs only contained the flowers that managed to use the morning fogs, called June Gloom by the locals, to stay alive despite the almost year since it had rained. Even in the plant world the only ones that adapted survived.

Don't cut it short he told himself: go all the way to the mile marker before turning around. Some days it seemed as if the wind was against him both coming and going. He followed his habit of looking at the cliffs on the way out and the ocean on the way back. The waves were too small today to be of interest to even the youngest of surfers. After glancing at the blue house and rounding the bend, he could see the finish line in the distance. He smiled at the baby plovers scampering back and forth with the crashing waves. The life guard stand was empty as it always was this time of year. He was too close to stop now. The next interim goal was the imaginary finish line and he visualized himself sprinting across this line in the sand with the determination and pride of a champion. His feet were now moving a little faster as he dashed past the big rock finish line. He slowed down his pace, walked for a short time and then stopped, putting his hands on his hips and looked around. He was all alone, having no one present to share the joy of this special moment; but he was OK with this. He smiled with the satisfaction that comes from achieving a challenging personal goal and was humbled as he realized that accomplishing goals was becoming a habit.

That man was me! I hope readers forgive me for writing of this experience in the third person but it enabled me to fully appreciate this otherwise indescribable emotional impact I experienced. At that moment, on that beach, I shook the sweat off my cap, gave thanks, stood a little taller, and walked back up those wooden steps resolving to address problems before they reached crisis mode. Had I had warning signs?

My history: In the couple of years prior to my demise, I had noticed that I would struggle to do the same physical activities I used to easily do. Relying on the clean bill of health from my physicians, I attributed my short comings to two things: age and being out of shape. I was aware that performance diminishes with age, so each time I was unable to do something, I didn't know whether to attribute it to age or being out-of-shape.

Were there any warning signs in the year before my heart stoppage? There was the time when I could not keep up with my daughter walking her dog around town, which I attributed to her habit of almost jogging over a somewhat hilly terrain. The sweat dripping off the visor of my ball cap bothered me on these warm days with moderate humidity. However, I always perspired profusely, and I did not experience any pain or discomfort.

While consulting, I remember going home for lunch one day as I felt so tired. I simply collapsed into my recliner and after an hour, I felt fine. After I stopped consulting, my daily routine of walking/jogging went smoothly but the elliptical machines at the YMCA were different. story. I could fight through the tiredness of moving both my arms and legs at the same time, but my heart rate would become worrisome. At rest my heart rate was 64 beats per minute. The chart on the machine indicated that my maximum rate was 140 for my age. The medical and sports advice was to increase my exercising rate to a maximum of 80% over resting rate, or 115 for me. Which was the norm for me? Discretion indicated that if in doubt, choose the lower one; but a good workout indicated the higher one. I decided that both numbers were generic estimates, so I would set my own. I noticed a pattern: for the first couple of minutes my heart rate would be in the 60s, then it moved slowly at first but once it reached 100 beats a minute, it escalated quickly. At about seven minutes into my exercise, when my heart rate would pass130, I would start to feel "strange." I would slow down until my heart rate dropped below 120 and if the strange feeling continued, I would stop and rest. I was proud of tripling my time on the elliptical machine to 24 minutes, and I believed my cardiologist who said there were no problems with my heart. Later I realized that the machine indicated a maximum rate of 140, and the target rate for exercise should have been 80% of 140 or 112.

One day I was shooting a basketball when a teenager, who was several inches taller and 50 pounds lighter, challenged me to a game of one-on-one. The sportsmanship in me accepted. I began by hitting a couple of outside shots and hung on by maneuvering, rather than running or jumping, and using my weight to keep him away from the basket. When my winning shot bounced in, I quickly declined a rematch, drove home, collapsed into my recliner and retired from competitive basketball: but I had no pains.

Over Thanksgiving we left sea level for a visit to Yosemite National Park; a beautiful park in the Sierra Nevada Mountains with altitudes between 2,000 and 13,000 feet. On a sunny, warm day while hiking with Carol up a gradual slope in a remote part of Yosemite, I had to slow down so much that I was being passed by very young children. Finally, with sweat dripping off me and feeling overwhelmingly weary, I sat on a log. I wanted to go on but this was the first time that I could not attribute my condition to my age or being out-of-shape. When I started wondering what would happen if I needed help, we headed back. I remember a little pressure but no pain. As a preventative measure, at home I saw a physician at Urgent Care who, while not finding anything wrong at sea level, suggested that I have another stress test "sooner rather than later." Thank you doctor! I scheduled a test for December 6, but on that day my 13-year old Jag failed to start, which caused me to reschedule the test to January 10.

On a warm, but not hot, day over Christmas, I went hiking with my daughter on a low trail in the Santa Ynez Mountains. She jogged up the first hill but only halfway up, I was sweating so heavily and felt so weary that I sat on a log under a tree and drank water. In a few minutes, feeling better, I stood and during the remainder of the hike, these symptoms did not reappear. Also over Christmas, I sweated profusely while playing golf and had no distance on my golf shots.

The American Heart Association (AHA): The following are the warning signs identified by AHA:

1.Chest Discomfort: usually in the center of the chest; lasts for a few minutes and can return; a feeling of uncomfortable pressure, squeezing, fullness or pain. I experienced strange feelings in my chest at Yosemite and the YMCA that I would describe as pressure, but not as a squeezing or pain. Apparently, I have a high threshold for pain, which is both a blessing and a curse. I rarely feel pain even when circumstances seem to indicate that I should. This sometimes causes me to mislead doctors when they ask me to rank my pain on a scale of 1-10, since I consider 10 to be death.

2. Discomfort: a pain or discomfort in other areas of the upper body; such as arms, back, neck, jaw, and stomach. I had no identifiable discomfort in other parts of my body.

3. Shortness of breath: I experienced shortness of breath but I mistakenly attributed it to age and/or being out-of-shape rather than a warning. I did have shortness of breath while walking and hiking.

4. Other Signs: breaking out in a cold sweat, nausea or light headiness. I profusely sweated but I always perspire profusely. The AHA symptom was described as "cold sweats" which is sweating not caused by heat or exertion, usually occurring at night (ask.me.com) which was not the case with me. I did not experience nausea or light headiness.

The AHA also indicates there may be some differences between men and women. Typical warning signs in men are chest pains, which are also a warning sign for women; although women are somewhat more likely to have other signs, such as shortness of breath, nausea/vomiting, and back or jaw pains.

Following the AHA recommendation of stopping the activities probably saved my heart so it could later be used for my second life.

Conclusion: Learning the AHA warning signs would have helped me along with taking more responsibility of my own health by listening to my body, rather than completely relying on my annual physical and stress test at the beginning of the year. Thank you Urgent Care doctor: had my Jag started, you may have prevented my crisis.

I did have some weariness and increases in my heart rate, but these symptoms are not on the AHA list. Also not on their list were any non-physical signs: were there any? The answer was a definite "yes," from multiple problems with my Delaware house, a family member, moving and renovating a condo. I concluded that stress was the culprit.

Stress for me is always involved, so I needed to monitor myself and be concerned with changes even if they did not exactly match the ones identified by the AHA, such as, do I feel tired for days? Am I looking at things negatively? Am I practicing "stress relievers?" If the situation does not improve, am I seeking help from a family member, friend, clergymen or professional?

Lessons Learned:

1. Take responsibility for your own life by learning the warning signs for heart problems and that symptoms may vary from person-to-person for a variety of reasons, such as age or gender. Know your body and listen to it.

2. Obtain the assistance of a medical team that, hopefully, already has a base line established for you.

3. Describe your feelings and concerns to your doctor even if you think the only causes are age or being out-of-shape.

4. Monitor the signs of stress, such as your attitude, relationship with others, physical activities, energy level and sleep pattern. Make appropriate changes as required to manage your stress level.

CHAPTER 28. JANUARY: THE CAUSE OF MY DEMISE

My feet barely touched the sand as they covered the short distance from the last interim goal to the magic finish line drawn by my mind. I did it! Nine days before my first birthday of my second life, I jogged the same distance I used to jog by the Brandywine River before my heart problems: three miles without stopping. I felt an indescribable joy. To be sure, jogging three miles was satisfying in and of itself. But it was even sweeter achieving a goal that had started as a dream. "A goal is a dream with a deadline" (Napoleon Hill).

January 1st had been selected as my "race day" so that the finish line could symbolize the finish of a tough year, and the beginning of a New Year and lifestyle. In a way, finishing was anti- climatic. My race really began the day after my heart surgery. Just being here, or for that matter being anywhere, meant I had already won the race to live.

Just a few hours before on New Year's Eve after celebrating my daughter's birthday, there were no new resolutions, no new "to do" lists: just a very humble thanks for being one of the three percent who after their heart stopped were given a second chance. For almost forty years, the words "second chance" instantly caused my stomach to knot over the dread that I felt when sitting in front of the desk of Dr. Clinton Whitehurst in his office in Sirrine Hall at Clemson University. He said, "Admitting me to the masters program had been a mistake. But it was my mistake as you had been honest with me. Mr. Zepke, few people are given a second chance in life, and even fewer take advantage of it. I hope you are one of them." Those words changed my life! I left his office determined to justify his hopes in me, as well as my own. I still remember the thrill when at the end of the semester, he awarded me a Stewart F. Brown Fellowship. Subsequently, it was his recommendation that enabled me to become a faculty member at The University of Tennessee, which then enabled me to finance my law school education that began my legal career. Every couple of years I sent him a note of thanks for that second chance.

On this New Year's Day, completing my goal was gratifying but not satisfying. Gratifying in that I now knew my one heart could support two lives and my "Managing Your (my) Rehabilitation Program WELL" was working, but to be satisfied I had to answer a key question.

Why had my heart stopped? While lying in Intensive Care that Saturday, I thought it might be my last day alive. I resolved that if I was given another "second" chance, I would learn what had caused me to be that desperate. During the ensuing year, my recovery had taken precedence. Now it was time to answer that question.

To put it simply, this question was just too important for me not to know. Obviously, I did something to cause my problems. My thoughts were captured in a forceful, yet articulate choice of words attributed to Albert Einstein, "Insanity is doing the same thing over and over and expecting different results." My humble choice of words was, "Until I know what I was doing wrong, how can I prevent starting the same cycle of destruction?"

Who was the right person to find the cause of my demise? The obvious answer was the cardiologist who had been treating me. However, even from my hospital bed, I had found his saying the cause was "the lack of potassium" was not credible. I had never had a potassium problem, and the blood test just three months prior indicated that I was within normal range for everything, including potassium (My new cardiologist subsequently confirmed that low potassium was the result, not the cause, of my heart stoppage).

My next question to the cardiologist was, "How did I pass the stress test if my arteries were so clogged?" His response of, "You did not pass." Whoa, I thought, what good would it do to wait until after my heart stopped before telling me that I had failed?" His explanation reminded me of the words of Supreme Court Justice Scalia, "The operation was a success, but the patient died," (*National Endowment for the Arts v. Finley*, 524 U.S. 569). I never anticipated using my skills as a lawyer in this situation, but habits honed over thirty years can be powerful.

My legal background was in gear when I asked, "What can I do to prevent my arteries from clogging again?" His response was, "Live a healthy life." If he were on the witness stand, I would have asked the judge to declare him a hostile witness (one who is antagonistic to the person asking the questions and/or is evasive). With a hostile witness, I could follow up with questions such as "That is a result, not a cause." But this was not a court of law, and my interest was in obtaining answers to the type of remedy not offered by courts: a healthy life. His answer made it obvious that he was not the appropriate person to ask: who was?

Was I the right person? My weaknesses were obvious: I was not a physician; much less a cardiac surgeon, cardiologist, vascular surgeon, pulmonologist or nurse. I had no hope of learning the medical vocabulary. I had not examined myself and the few tests results available to me did not indicate any blockages.

My strengths were much less obvious. My lack of medical training and vocabulary could also be a plus as mine were a "fresh pair of eyes" that would question everything and not get distracted from the concepts by vocabulary words and industry jargon. There was another qualification that was unique to me. I was the only person who could say, "Everywhere I went, there I was." No one else had "walked in my moccasins." While I certainly would not have volunteered to be the one to have undergone my experiences, perhaps it was fortuitous for other patients that they happened to someone experienced in both quantitatively analyzing events, as well as in presenting them in a way that could be understood by juries.

My inquiries had really started in that hospital bed on the day before my heart surgery when I had reviewed my life searching for one or more destructive habits. It was not a time to sugar coat anything, which was why I did not duck the pre-op nurse's question about out-of-body experiences.

A first-person, post mortem investigation? My research would have another aspect that made it unique; so unique that it probably never had been done before, nor would ever be done again. I was going to conduct a first-person, post-mortem investigation. Some folks may be able to write about potential problems, or close calls, but almost no one could help others by writing a first-person, post mortem account.

I no longer questioned that my heart stopped because it got out of rhythm, which to me meant that the blood did not move through the chambers in the expected volume and velocity. This disrupted the timing and "confused," "overwhelmed" or whatever is the appropriate verb, the "timing mechanism" for my heart, and it stopped. I reasoned that my heart stopped during the stress echo test due to the very stress the test was designed to create. The cause of my heart straining was my clogged arteries. However, in the year since I had passed the same stress test, had the blockage in my arteries progressed to the point of causing the crisis or were one of the two stress tests in error?

My inquiry became "If the test results the year prior were correct, then what I had done to so clog my arteries in just one year? If the previous year's test results were incorrect, then I needed to look at my habits over a much greater time period. So the question was: were the results of the 2006 test correctly interpreted?

The Analysis: The stress test uses an electrocardiogram to measure the rhythm of hearts both at rest and when stressed. It is so widely used that it is doubtful that the test is faulty. However, it is calibrated to only indicate a problem when an artery is clogged more than 70%. For example, if a patient's three arteries were clogged anywhere from zero to close to, but less than 70%, they would pass the stress echo test. I was told that I passed the test in 2006, which would indicate that all three of my arteries were clogged less than 70%.

In 2007 the same stress echo test not being stopped indicated that either the test did not identify a significant blockage, or it did and the operators missed it. The actual measurements of my blockage were 80%, 90% and 100%.

The results of the analysis using the Chi Square statistical model was that the probability of the 2006 test being correct was much less than 1%! So much less as to be approaching an impossibility. Put into plain English, the results of the 2006 test had to be erroneous.

Was the error in the test or the interpretation?

It was highly unlikely that a test so widely used by the medical profession could provide errors of this magnitude, so the 2006 test results were not properly interpreted. A proper interpretation could have led to procedures to prevent the heart stopping crisis.

Did my analysis convert my gratification to satisfaction? It proved that it was a human error that contributed to the necessity for "One Heart – Two Lives" by not identifying my blockage in 2006, or by stopping the test in 2007 before my heart stopped. However, since all exams and tests are administered by people, even well trained, dedicated, caring people make mistakes as "people are human" (Krugman, NY Times, 2/14/2012). Diagnosing my blockage earlier would have prevented my one heart from having to serve two lives, but why had my arteries been so blocked?

The potential causes listed by the American Heart Association are:

Genes – NOT a factor, mine were great.

Smoking – N OT a factor; I never smoked.

Exercise – NOT a factor as I was exercising regularly.

Diet – NOT a factor based on my BMI.

Cholesterol – NOT a factor as it was close to normal.

Stress – The only measurement I was aware of was blood pressure, and mine was a little high, but not high enough for physicians to prescribe pills. Still, I felt this was a problem not only because I had eliminated all other possible causes, but also because it was the one that for years I had been unable to control.

Stress and blocked arteries? How could stress be related to blocked arteries? I understood that genes have a great impact on our internal compositions; smoking and diet to what we force our bodies to process; and exercise to how it is processed. But how did stress fit in?

I understood that stress may cause people to do certain physical things. For example, while studying for the bar exam, I gained 17 pounds in six weeks. The theoretical question was confusing but coming at the question another way helped. People under stress have much higher incidents of every imaginable malady. I wasn't sure why but since every part of our body is dependent on the other parts doing their jobs, a break down anywhere may well cause failures elsewhere. I would try to improve the way I handled stress.

Responsibility: This was painful reminder that the ultimate responsibility for my health rests with me! I made some poor decisions, such as not scheduling the test sooner, and a few great ones, like stopping my exercises whenever I felt "funny." I wonder how many of those times saved my life?

Medical professionals are all humans, and no humans are perfect, or to paraphrase a quote I remember from high school "To err is human; to forgive, divine" (Alexander Pope, 1688-1744). That I am here and able to write this is a testimony to the large number of caring medical professionals who helped me. That said, I still needed to take responsibility to become a better educated patient and be more pro-active in questioning any procedure, medication or treatment. I also had to do a better job of identifying and communicating any potential warning signs.

Conclusion: While jogging my subconscious produced an epitome, had I asked the right question for heart patients? I thought the key question "what was the cause of my demise" but when I learned the answer, I realize my mistake. The answer was helpful in that it led to my changing those habits. While this was "gratifying," it was "satisfying," because to be satisfying the question had to be "how could I prevent future heart problems?" When I realized that the cause of any future heart problems might not be the same as ones for my previous problems, I realized that the cardiologist was right: I needed "To live a healthy lifestyle."

Lessons Learned:

Were there other signs, such as the reverse sequence of rehabilitating, in this sequence: (5) Reduced self actualization, such as my stopping the active practice of law; (4) reduced self worth, such as stopping practicing laws along with the decline in investments; (3) reduced social contacts, such as my leaving all my friends to move thousands of miles to a town where I knew only one person; (2) reduced security and safety, such as the destruction of my house and the theft of my possessions; (1) reduced physiological, such as the breakdown of my heart, not from a particular stimulus, but from the accumulated stress over many years.

CHAPTER 29. GOALS FOR TODAY & TOMORROW

"Managing Your (my) Rehabilitation Program WELL," successfully brought my "One Heart-Two Lives" through a tumultuous rehabilitation!

Cumulating the probabilities of the sequence starting with my heart stopping indicates that I was the one person in approximately one hundred million people to have my experiences. I will be eternally grateful for all the great people, guided by a hand from above, who enabled me to have the exciting luxury (as in comfort, delight, bliss, and sense of well being) of feeling this gratification.

Early in my rehabilitation, I decided that in order to prevent restarting the same behavior cycle over again, I would take the extra effort – although I had no idea how difficult this would be – to review my values and renew or create habits that re-enforced them. This was when gratification met satisfaction.

After a brief summary of my attitudinal progress, I will discuss how to create a system to continue using the principles of my book to create a user friendly, personal accountability system to establish habits that re-enforce your goals, which will convert gratification into satisfaction.

I noticed a pattern that could provide a guide for successfully "Managing Your Rehabilitation Program WELL" which, I believe, could also be helpful for patients rehabilitating from any malady, as well as their caregivers. An important caveat is that this guide is meant to supplement, not replace, the services and advice of skilled professionals.

The first step was physiological, which means establishing a physical structure for the journey from rehabilitation-to-recovery. To be a proactive teammate to the medical professions, rather than feeling like a helpless victim, focus on solutions which may help, and certainly would not hurt, the outcome (Chapter 6).

The second step was providing the safety and security of continued health care, shelter, food and clothing. After medical professionals have created a physical framework for rehabilitation, other caregivers, such as family, friends, counselors or trainers and even employers, can play an increased role (Chapter 14). But I would learn time and time again the steps of the rehab ladder were slippery and may require a step back down, such as when our income and healthcare were threatened by a bank employee (Chapter 22).

The third step was rebuilding my social world, meaning my interactions with family, friends and colleagues. The importance of the social aspects were illustrated by the Stockholm Syndrome where people were reluctant to terminate even harmful social relationships.

The fourth step was re-establishing my feelings of self worth or, phrased differently, self-esteem, which is the confidence of achievement and the accompanying respect by myself and others.

The fifth step was self-actualization, which is growing through our values towards achieving our potentials.

Attitude: My research into how to handle stress led me to the quote of "Grant me the courage to change the things I can change, the serenity to accept the things I can't change, and the wisdom to know the difference" (Reinhold Niebuhr, American theologian, 1892-1971), which the American Psychological Association (APA) identified as "perhaps the best general approach for treating stress" (reutershealth.com).

Like many people, I was aware of this quote, but when my stress forced me into "Managing Your (my) Rehabilitation Program WELL," I started to "have the courage to change the things I can change." It began with my developing a better understanding of my physical condition so I could safely expand it (rehabilitation; Voldyne; lung surgery; Las Vegas; flying to, and meetings in, New York) and defend it (Mazatlan). My next steps were to develop a better understanding of myself by reviewing my values and habits to determine which ones should be changed.

In a much humbler way, my small world during rehabilitation provided an environment conducive to increasing my understandings of myself, my surroundings and my place in it – much the same way that Henry David Thoreau used his two years besides Walden's Pond and Wyeth who lived in the rural Brandywine River Valley and Maine. Thoreau very eloquently used his writings, and Andrew Wyeth equally used his paintings, to indicate the "serenity of accepting" the undraped beauty of things, and persons, that surround us.

The beach, by reducing distractions, became my version of Thoreau's pond and Wyeth's Brandywine River. "Changing the things I can change" was illustrated by creating the habit of jogging while paying more attention to my surroundings. The beauty and roles played by inanimate objects, like rocks and kelp, re-enforced the "serenity of accepting the things I can't change." The spirit of the living things continuing with their lives despite limiting circumstances (a wounded seal lying on the beach, a three-legged dog guarding its master, or the Great Dane trying to please its master while declining a little more each day) re-enforced the "wisdom to know the difference."

An exciting part of wanting to not just return to my condition before my heart stopped, but to improve on it. This is what caused me to review my values and habits, which stimulated an increased awareness and appreciation of my surrounding environment: now that was exciting!

Goals: Use the Manage Annual Plans or MAP system (discussed in Chapter 26) to create habits to implement your values through annual goals. To implement the MAP system, I wrote a one page annual plan setting forth my goals at the beginning of each year.

Your responsibilities: We are all ultimately responsible for our lives, including our health with no exceptions! The medical community can, and must, be a vital resource. But please learn from my example that despite having annual physicals, including blood work and being in the care of a cardiologist, my heart stopped. This is not to indicate that physicians do not do a great job: they do! In fact without a terrific sequence of surgeons, I would not be enjoying my second life. Rather it is the recognition that they are people with the ever-increasing demands of the practice of medicine. The following are some specific things I will use to control and monitor my health.

Stress: When I stopped seeking perfection in everything, my

stress dropped. I will be alert for excessive stresses, such as after the death of a loved one, divorce, loss of job, increased financial obligations, getting married, moving, chronic injury or illness, emotional problems, taking care of family member, and traumatic events (Web.MD), which may cause changes in my habits – temperament, physical routines, manner of dress – or my words or social interactions for potential indicators.

Physical: I will continue to have annual physicals where I will pay more attention to the details of medical reports and tests and follow up with any relevant specialist (cardiologist and now dermatologist, as I already have had skin cancer), including keeping my medical team current. Regular exercise and taking my prescriptions will put me in the upper 30% of preventative care since 70% of heart patients do not take even these minimum preventative measures!

The speakers in rehab stimulated me to sometimes visualize my stomach as a cartoon character saying, "Now what does he expect us to do with this stuff he just swallowed?" As entertaining as this was, it also triggered my thinking of my body as having to process everything by either burning it as energy, passing it as waste or storing it as fat.

Metabolism, or the basal "metabolic rate," is the process by which we convert food and drink into energy for breathing, circulating blood, hormone levels and growing and repairing cells. The food and drink not converted is either expelled or stored as fat. In general, metabolism is greater in males than females, greater in lean muscular bodies and decreases 5% for each decade we age after 40. Metabolism may be partly responsible for gaining weight, along with our inherited genetics, hormonal controls and our lifestyle choices of sleep, physical activity and stress (Mayo Clinic).

Exercise is vitally important in maintaining good health. Heart patients (and others) should consult experts before beginning either cardiovascular or resistance exercises. My rehab program provided a safe start for the cardiovascular by creating the habit of slowly increasing the pace and/or distance, like I did for my jogging. My rule of thumb is at least a half hour of cardio exercise five times a week. There are many helpful forms of yoga that provide instructions on techniques of stretching and breathing. Resistance training helps slow down the natural loss of muscle that occurs past 60.

Diet: Besides the experts, there are many great sources for selecting good diets, such as the American Dietetic Association (eatright.org), Health Information (melineplus.gov) and Health and Nutrition (webmd.com). My formal rehab program recommended to decrease saturated trans fatty acids, total fats and cholesterol. Increase Omega 3 fats and foods made from soy. Choose unrefined carbohydrates with fiber.

In restaurants, I no longer use salt (it raises blood pressure) and pay more attention to ingredients, particularly appetizers and desserts, and avoid or choose substitutes for unhealthy dishes. I eat most things in moderation and chew slowly to better taste the food and to provide time for my stomach to indicate when it is full.

Liquids: I drink water although I found the recommended 64 ounces a day too laborious, so I drink at least one big glass of water at every meal, which has the added benefit of making me eat less. I drink three cups of coffee, although green tea is preferable, and a glass or two of wine. The National Institute of Alcohol Abuse (NIAAA) indicates the probability of health abuse is low for men who have no more than 14 drinks a week (7 for women), and some studies indicate that people who drink at that level have a lower risk of cardiovascular disease, depression and some cognitive issues than those who don't drink any alcohol.

Cholesterol, one of many substances created and used by our bodies to keep us healthy, is also found in foods from animal sources such as meat, poultry and full-fat dairy products. Experts recommend men over 35 and women over 40 have a "lipid profile" done every couple of years (WebMD) to measure your types of cholesterol. The low density protein cholesterol (LDL) is called the "bad" one because it can build up in the walls of your arteries and, if it breaks loose, cause a stroke or heart attack (American Heart Association). The high density cholesterol (HDL) is called the "good" one because it tends to reduce the negative effects of LDL. The listed standards (including triglycerides which carry fats in the blood) are:

Total of LDL and HDL in mg/dl	category	Triglycerides
Less than 200	desirable	less than 150
200-239	borderline high	150-190
240+	high	200-499

Heart rate is important to monitor but discussions of heart rates can be complex. Interested persons should contact a professional for their specific situation. To take your heart rate, referred to "pulse" rate, (1) use the tips of your first two fingers to lightly press the vein on the thumb side of one of your wrists and (2) count your pulse rate for 10 seconds and multiply by 6 to obtain your rate per minute. The National Institute of Health (NIH) provides that the average "resting" heart rate for anyone over 10 years old is 60-100 beats per minute. For well-trained athletes, it is 40-60.

For the "maximum" heart rate while exercising, the NIH recommends subtracting your age from 220. For example, my maximum heart rate at age 63 was 220-63=157 beats per minute.

For a "target" range while exercising, the NIH recommends between 50% and 80% of my maximum rate. Based on my maximum rate of 157, the calculations would be 50% of 157= 79 and 85% of 157=133, so my target zone for exercise was between 79-133 beats per minute. In general the greater the rate the more energy burned.

There are other methods to target heart rate while exercising with the ultimate test being how you feel. Stopping when I did not feel quite right probably saved my life!

Blood pressure, like heart rate, should be discussed with medical professionals as it can change with postures, exercise, stress or sleep. The guidelines of the American Heart Association are as follows:

	Systolic	Diastolic
Pre-hypertension	120-139	80-89
Stage 1 HBP	140-159	90-99
Stage 2 HBP	160 and higher	100 and higher
Crisis HBP	higher than 180	higher than 110

Systolic increases with age due to stiffness of arteries, build-up of plaque and cardiac and vascular disease. My experience was that my pressure was always in the pre-hypertension range so my physicians recommended changes in my diet and exercise program.

Now besides taking blood pressure pills, I do a better job of monitoring myself with a home machine (I recommend checking its accuracy by having a professional check against their results).

Weight is important to control as too much weight tends to

increase the risk of many problems, such as heart-related ones. The recommended standard is the Body Mass Index (BMI), which is approved by the National Heart, Lung and Blood Institute (NHLBI). Enter your height and weight on the BMI chart (nhibi.nih.gov) to obtain a corresponding BMI number:

> 18.5 or less is underweight;
> 18.5-24.9 is normal;
> 25-29.9 is overweight;
> 30 or greater is obese.

Having a large body frame and muscle weighing more than fat may provide a little leeway. A caveat is that BMI does not measure the fat in arteries.

Conclusion: My wish to share the thrill of hearing your love one (in my case my daughter) say, 'Dad, we are sorry you had a heart problem, but if you had to have one, we wish you had it years ago," was a tremendous motivating factor in my undertaking the laborious writing task of sharing my approach through this book.

I hope readers learn as much from reading this book as I did from writing it. It has been said that "Every man is the builder of a temple called his body. We are sculptors, painters, and our material is our flesh and blood and bones" (Ralph Waldo Emerson). Hopefully my sharing my approach as a "thoughtful" builder, sculptor and painter will illustrate a potential path to avoid a heart crisis or, if one occurs, for you to join me in using the opportunities discussed in *One Heart-Two Lives: Managing Your Rehabilitation Program WELL.*

APPENDIX 1
CHAPTER 30: CAREGIVERS

The moisture filling my eyes would have made me think I was crying except that men don't cry. It wasn't that I hurt any more than yesterday: I did not. It wasn't a specific event: there weren't any. It wasn't because I was a heart patient: I was thrilled to have a second chance at life. It was a tear of frustration and helplessness. Frustration, a feeling of being upset or annoyed at an inability to change or achieve something, can be that way. Helplessness as day-by-day I watched my wife give as much as she could for as long as she could until she started moving a little slower, looking a little wearier and talking a little slower as her energies slowly lost their battle with her fatigue. The "tears" were from recognizing, but not only being able to stop the increasing demands of her 50+ hour work week, but also from my being helpless to reduce needing her help full time.

So I sat there like a helpless child with the difference being I recognized the symptoms and all I could do was hope that her energies would outlast my needs. I later learned I was not alone in these feelings.

Millions of caregivers: The U.S. Center for Disease Control (CDC) complied some statistics on caregivers, including:

    - There are more than 34 million unpaid caregivers (approximately the population of Canada) providing care for someone age 18, and older, who has an illness of disability.

    -The majority (83%), or 28 million, are unpaid family caregivers, such as family members, relatives or neighbors.

- Caregivers report having trouble finding time for themselves (35%), managing emotional and physical stress (29%) and balancing work and family responsibilities (29%).

- More than half (51%) said they do not have time to take care of themselves and almost half are too tired to do so.

- Half (53%), or 18.02 million (approximately the population of Florida) said their health had gotten worse due to caregiving also said the decline in their health affected their ability to provide care.

There are tens of millions of caregivers in all of these categories.

Personal experiences: In the hospital there is a trained, dedicated, full-time, paid and unpaid, team of caregivers that assist patients in many ways (providing encouragement, understanding and, for me, even from coming out of the anesthetic too soon). My experience was similar to the statistics that indicated even after discharge, a heart patient can need a caregiver, perhaps even full time.

In our case I sat there helplessly day after day watching my caregiver/wife talk into the headset while stealing caring glances at me in-between key strokes into the ever present laptop. Our need for her income required that we gamble that one of her two full-time duties broke before she did! What a thing to gamble with!

Watching her stirred up a kaleidoscope of feelings that were unceasingly vying for dominance. I had been caregiver for my wife Anne, and our three children under ten, as she bravely fought, and lost, her three-year battle with cancer. No matter what I did, I felt guilty at what I was not doing. When I was earning sufficient income a thousand miles away, I worried about not being with my family. When I returned home without a job, I worried about how to support them. When I was employed at a much lesser job an hour away, I worried about both not being there and supporting them.

On the mornings when my arms would feel so heavy that I had to reach for the energy to shave, I would say to myself, "Come on Brent, you can stand on your head all day if necessary. How can you think of yourself when Anne is fighting for her life and your children need you?" Determination, less sleep and more coffee got me through most days. I knew I was in trouble the time I came in my front door at 7 P.M. thinking, "I have to hurry as I have to leave for work in less than 12 hours," and the time I was standing in my doorway trying to remember whether I was coming from, or going to, work. This was exactly the midpoint of the 20-25 years cardiologists indicate that is typical for a buildup of plaque in arteries.

The stress of always trying to do more, or as I came to think of it, being "A man for all seasons," (from the book of the same name by Robert Bolt), came to a head the day I crashed with the thought that "superman died." For years afterwards, I was haunted by thoughts that I could have done more if only I'd known how.

Now I saw some of the same signs of stress in Carol. She would sound apologetic when she had to leave our condo to go her office or the grocery store. I even watched her tend to her nails with a cell phone propped against her shoulder since the conversation was too confidential for her to use a headset or speaker.

Threats to caregivers: Caregivers can put aside their own needs day-to-day but the accumulation increases the risks of caregivers becoming patients. One graphic personal example of my role changing occurred after I slept on a cot at the foot of Anne's hospital bed in the oncology ward. In the morning my back spasms forced me to roll over the side and kneel on the floor. This hospital did not have an orthopedic department, so I hobbled to the lobby, took a cab to another hospital, hobbled into the emergency room and after popping pain pills and muscle relaxers, I returned: I was 40.

However, whether the caregiver is 8 or 80, the threat is the same: to stay vertical and healthy enough to be able to continue for a day, week, month or whatever it takes. The CDC's statistics indicate that millions of caregivers have difficulty in being able to continue functioning as a person and, secondarily, to give care to family members where the caregiver is the primary wage earner.

The CDC indicates there are 28 million unpaid family caregivers. In the Mended Hearts *Heartbeat* Magazine, some family caregivers expressed their greatest challenges as (1) watching your vibrant love one go through all the physical and mental strain, (2) accepting the limitations that a heart patient faces, (3) finding the time to care for themselves, (4) not knowing if they will recognize signs of heart failure, (5) feeling guilty by not doing enough or taking time to pursue their own interests, and (6) the panic of not knowing what the future will hold or whether there will even be a future. My experience was that the longer they existed for my caregiver, Carol, the greater her physical and mental challenges would become.

Tips for Caregivers include:

- Take care of yourself so you will be able to continue being a caregiver and not a care receiver.
- Get organized by writing things down in lists and keeping it handy for whenever someone else asks what they can do to help.
- Keep medical records and a list of medications handy.
- Organize bills and review monthly.
- Keep a notebook handy and write down questions as you think of them and seek answers.
- Taking breaks from caretaking duties increases your performance and productivity.
- See your physician regularly.
- Follow the same guidelines for patients to eat and drink healthy foods and beverages, while fighting the temptation to consume copious cups of coffee and unhealthy snacks.
- Get cardiovascular exercise at least twenty minutes a day even if it is a brisk walk around a hospital.
- Maintain your normal social contacts and stay active in family activities.
- Keep some hobbies or other distractions as a way to take a mental vacation; keeping your hands busy may help.

Sources for additional information and assistance:

- Mended Hearts (1-888-HEART-99, mendedheart.org)
- National Alliance for Caregivers (NAC)
- Institute for Medicine (IOM)
- Family Caregiver Alliance (FCA)

APPENDIX 2
CHAPTER 31. POST-TRAUMATIC STRESS DISORDER AND HEART PROBLEMS

Post Traumatic Stress Disorder (PTSD), which was first brought to the publics' attention by war veterans, can actually result from any number of tragic events that threatens a person's life. For example, studies now indicate that a significantly high percentage of heart patients may develop PTSD (Columbia University study, NY Times, June 20, 2012). This important topic is included as an appendix because, unlike the rest of the book, it is not written from a first person basis.

Heart patients statistics: For heart patients the numbers are significant. The Columbia University study stated there are 1.4 million patients discharged from a hospital each year after a heart attack or other coronary event. This is equivalent to having every person in our fifth largest city, Philadelphia, discharged from a hospital every year after a heart attack or other coronary event. Of the 1.4 million, 168,000 will develop "clinically significant" symptoms of PTSD; the equivalent of having every person in Chattanooga, Tennessee, or Sydney, Australia, suffering from PTSD after being released from being hospitalized for heart problems. The 168,000 out of 1.4 million is equivalent to 12%, or 1 in every 8 heart patients discharged after heart problems experiencing clinically significant PTSD. This 12% is 900% higher than the estimated 1.3% of the general population suffering from clinically significant PTSD. For these heart patients, the risk of dying within 2-3 years doubled (Columbia University study).

PTSD: An estimated 3.5% of the entire U.S. adult population suffers some symptoms of PTSD (The National Institute of Mental Health (NIMH)). PTSD, which was once referred to as "battle fatigue" or "shell shock," is a debilitating condition that typically follows a terrifying event. It can consist of a physical weakness and mental symptoms. Often people with PTSD have persistent and frightening thoughts of their ordeal and may feel emotionally numb. It can be caused by any traumatic incident, which could be anything that threatens the person's life or the life of someone close, or witnessing an act of mass destruction, like a plane crash. Some examples are violent attacks, such as a mugging, rape, torture, kidnapping or being held captive. The lynch pin is the person feeling threatened and experiencing feelings of intense fear, helplessness or horror.

Not every traumatized person will get PTSD, but for those who do, it varies in severity. My personal experience was that the issue was not whether people with heart problems feel threatened and experience fear, helplessness or horror: they do! The question was whether the level of intensity reaches a critical point, which is defined as becoming "clinically significant."

Diagnosing: Experts diagnose PTSD only after the symptoms last for more than a month. For heart patients the crucial time to watch for symptoms is within three months of the heart problem, although there have been cases where the illness did not show up until years later. If diagnosed and treated in its early stage before it becomes severe, it can save a life. The course of the illness varies as some people recover within six months while others may have symptoms that last much longer, including becoming chronic.

Clinically significant: "Clinically significant" PTSD has been defined as "significant distress or impairment in social, occupational or other important areas of functioning" (John Cannell, MD). While 3.5% of the population have some symptoms, only 1.3% have clinically significant symptoms while 12% of discharged heart patients have them (Columbia University study).

The general symptoms include having difficulty sleeping, being irritable, outbursts of anger, difficulty concentrating, hyper-vigilance, or exaggerated or startled responses. If these symptoms adversely impact the person's functioning or are resulting in significant distress, they may be clinically significant.

"Clinically significant" is defined as a person having at least one clinically significant symptom of (A) re-experiencing the event and (B) at least three clinically significant symptoms of avoidance or emotional numbing (American Psychiatric Association).

A. Re-experiencing the event can occur in one or more of the following ways (for clinically significant need at least one of these):

1. Recurring recollections of the event, including images, thoughts or perceptions.

2. Recurrent distressing dreams of the event.

3. Acting or feeling the event is recurring, including those that occur while intoxicated.

4. Intense psychological distress at exposure to internal or external cues that symbolize the event.

5. Physiological reactivity on exposure to internal or external cues that symbolize or resemble an aspect of the traumatic event.

All five of these could be threatening to the person's security and 3 and 4 can impact them physiologically. "Recurring" is the nexus of the symptoms of "re-experiencing" the event that makes it fit the definition of a habit. If a patient creates a habit of discussing, in a distressed way, their heart attack or surgery, they may have the symptoms of the first part of the test.

B. Avoidance or emotional numbing symptoms (for clinically significant need at least 3 of these) are:

1. Efforts to avoid conversations associated with the trauma.

2. Efforts to avoid activities, places or people that arouse recollections of the event.

3. Inability to recall an important aspect of the trauma.

4. Diminished interest in significant activities.

5. Feeling detached or estranged from others.

6. Restricted range of affections.

7. A sense of not being able to have a career, marriage, children or normal life span.

In the hierarchy of needs, all but numbers 3 and 7 could be threatening to the social needs and 7 to self-worth. Number 3 might be related to blocking out memories of physical threats. The second part of the test involves patients creating new habits to avoid social contacts, including but not limited to those associated with their heart problem.

Many heart patients experience some of the symptoms. For example, it has been stated that one in five patients after heart surgery, or one in three patients after a heart attack, have a fantasy about dying (U.S. News.com). This may be stressful but it may not be PTSD where the symptoms typically appear within three months of the trauma.

 Recognizing and Treating PTSD: How can a heart patient, or a caregiver, recognize PTSD? The first part of the test involves identifying a habit of the patient focusing on the event of the heart problem. The second part of the test involves identifying a habit of avoidance of discussing the event, or showing affection, planning for the future, or being anxious around unfamiliar people or unfamiliar environments (American Association Nurses Anesthetists Journal December 2012).

The treatment depends on the severity. In severe cases, professional help should be sought. The traditional treatment is behavior therapy and anti- depressants. In most cases the PTSD will last one to six months. Since the symptoms can be classified under the needs hierarchy, caregivers might use this tool to meet their care receiver's security or physiological needs. Please remember that PTSD can be serious and should be handled with caution and care.

Things to do:

1. Understand that while most heart patients will not have clinically significant PTSD, some will resulting in danger of a much shorter life span unless treated by a medical professional.

2. Pay attention to patterns of conversations, particularly those involving the events surrounding the heart problem.

3. Encourage the patient to discuss the trauma, feelings or future plans.

4. Encourage the heart patient who is showing signs of PTSD to seek medical treatment immediately.

ABOUT THE AUTHOR

Brent E. Zepke, Esq., has written five nonfiction books and twenty articles on legal and business subjects. He was a faculty member at universities and conferences while practicing law for thirty years. He has a bachelor's degree in mathematics from the University of North Carolina, a masters degree in industrial management from Clemson University, a law degree from The University of Tennessee and an advanced law degree in labor law from Temple University.